COLLINS GEM
CATS
a mine of information

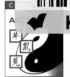

COLLINS GEM
A
牛
鼠
兔
a mine of information

KT-522-985

a mine of information

a mine of information

COLLINS GEM
HORSES
& PONIES
a mine of information

COLLINS GEM
INSECTS
a mine of information

COLLINS GEM
KINGS &
QUEENS
a mine of information

COLLINS GEM
MUSHROOMS
& TOADSTOOLS
a mine of information

COLLINS GEM
SNAKES
a mine of information

COLLINS GEM
SPIDERS
a mine of information

COLLINS GEM
STRESS
Survival Guide
a mine of information

COLLINS GEM
TAROT
a mine of information

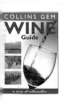

COLLINS GEM
WINE
Guide
a mine of information

COLLINS GEM
WORLD
atlas
a mine of information

COLLINS GEM
YOGA
a mine of information

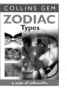

COLLINS GEM
ZODIAC
Types
a mine of information

COLLINS GEM

KEEPING FIT

Anne Charlish

HarperCollins*Publishers*

Anne Charlish is a medical and health writer and broadcaster. She has written more than 20 books and regularly contributes to leading women's magazines.

HarperCollins Publishers
PO Box, Glasgow G4 0NB

First published 1999

Reprint 10 9 8 7 6 5 4 3 2 1 0

Picture credits: Jan Croot, Ulrike Preuss,
Marcella Haddad, EMPICS
With thanks to the staff of Brixton Recreation Centre

ISBN 0 00 4722305-8

Printed in Italy by Amadeus S.p.A.

Contents

CONTENTS

FIT FOR LIFE
General fitness

Most of us would like to feel healthy and invigorated all of the time. The depressing feelings of sluggishness and lack of energy – such as after an illness or as a result of too many late nights – are something we would all like to avoid. One of the aims of this book is to provide knowledge about the basics of fitness.

HOW IS FITNESS DEFINED?

General fitness has several components:

- Muscular strength
- Muscular endurance
- Cardiovascular endurance
- Flexibility
- Speed
- Power

WHY DO I NEED TO BE FIT?

When we are fit, we manage all our everyday tasks in our work lives and our home lives with increased vitality and enthusiasm and reduced stress. We are much less likely to lose our temper under pressure if we are fit, or to make mistakes. We are more likely to enjoy our work and our family life and friendships.

YOU'RE UNFIT WHEN . . .

- You find it a struggle to reach the top of four flights of stairs
- You are out of breath after hurrying for a train
- You can't keep up with your young children
- You feel exhausted after an unusually strenuous game of tennis or badminton
- You drive everywhere
- You are gaining a little weight every year, year after year
- You become tired more easily than you used to

WHAT ARE THE PHYSICAL AND MENTAL ADVANTAGES OF GOOD GENERAL FITNESS?

Being fit helps to prevent heart disease and osteoporosis, controls blood pressure and diabetes, develops body strength, alleviates arthritis, improves mobility, reduces breathlessness on exertion and keeps your weight in check. It also helps you to fight off depression and feelings of apathy, reduces the risk of a stroke – which could leave you completely incapacitated – and reduces general everyday stress.

SOUNDS FAMILIAR?

You are probably not as fit as you would like to be or as fit as you need to be for your work and your lifestyle.

Doctors and other experts now recognize, unequivocally, that exercise and activity are good for us, both mentally and physically. They also know that many people are resistant to the idea of exercise for a variety of reasons:

- 'I can't find the time'
- 'It's all I can do, when I get home, to get the supper and collapse in front of the TV'
- 'I'm too old now'
- 'I'm always on my feet anyway – I certainly don't need to do any more'

THE TIME FACTOR

Take a good look at how you spend your evenings. Do you find time to watch something on TV when you could be exercising? Do you chat on the phone even though you know you are going to see that person at the weekend? What in your evenings or weekends can be relinquished to make space for half an hour's physical activity each day?

THE FATIGUE FACTOR

It is well known that regular exercise actually provides you with more energy rather than less. You won't believe it until you have actually done it, however. Try just once going for a walk after work, or going for a swim, and then see how much better you feel. You will also find that your quality of sleep is improved, so that you feel better when you wake up the next morning. Alternatively, go for a walk or a swim before work. You will find getting up half an hour earlier each morning reaps handsome rewards.

THE AGE FACTOR

Everyone, no matter what age, can benefit from activity. Nothing ages a person as fast as doing nothing. The more you do, the more you can do.

THE SUFFICIENCY-QUALITY FACTOR

Activity needs to be rhythmic and sustained to promote good general fitness. Rushing about at work or looking after a family is not likely to build up good fitness levels.

How do I achieve fitness?

There are six fundamental questions that need to be resolved if you are going to achieve and maintain fitness.

1 What do I do?

2 Where do I go?

3 What do I need in terms of equipment and clothing?

4 How long will it take before I notice a difference in my fitness levels?

5 What if I'm ill and inactive for a week or more – how do I regain lost fitness?

6 How can I find the time?

These are the questions that this book aims to answer.

ACHIEVING FITNESS

Question 1: What do I do?

Many experts believe that walking and swimming are the two best possible forms of exercise to undertake on a regular basis for optimum general fitness. They are both rhythmic and sustained and they both use several sets of muscles. Swimming uses nearly all the muscles of the body and is particularly suitable for very overweight, pregnant and elderly people because the weight of the body is borne by the water.

However, the activity that you choose is a matter of personal preference. Section II of this book describes the many options available to you.

You don't even need to go out of the house to achieve fitness: if the only way that you can manage 30 minutes' moderately brisk activity a day is to set aside the time at home, then choose from step exercises, walking up and downstairs, exercising with weights, skipping, sit ups, aerobics (to video or music), or stretch 'n' tone exercises – all of which are described in Section II.

Questions 2 and 3 are answered with each individual activity described in Section II.

Question 4: How long do I need to exercise to achieve good general fitness?

To maintain health you should exercise every day for 30 minutes. To build up and maintain fitness you should exercise for 30–60 minutes at an intensity of 60–90% of your maximum heart rate (see pp 60–61), on three to five days of the week, using any form of rhythmic, sustained activity.

Question 5: Regaining lost fitness

The only way is slowly but surely. Start with half an hour twice a week. Then, as you increase in fitness and confidence, increase to three times a week until you feel ready to exercise for half an hour five times a week. See also Fitness in later life on pp 52–57.

Question 6: The time factor

This depends a lot upon your personal motivation. If you really want to become fit (or fitter still), you will undoubtedly find the time – even if it means deciding that something in your life has to go, or be better organized:

- sheets, pillowcases, towels and underwear do not need to be ironed

- video your favourite TV programme in order to watch it later or at the weekend

- get up half an hour earlier in the morning

- forego that last drink in the pub

Body types

The human body has for many years been classified into
three main types: ectomorph, endomorph and
mesomorph. The ectomorph body tends to be lean and
wiry and not noticeably muscular. Ectomorphs are
notable for their endurance and agility and hence make
good cross-country runners. The endomorph body has
a soft, rounded appearance, and although suited to most
forms of exercise, endomorphs are advised to
concentrate on less strenuous activities. The mesomorph
body is stocky and usually well-muscled. The muscular
frame is capable of developing strength, endurance,
power and agility.

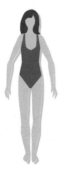
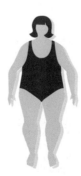
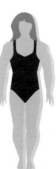

*The lean
ectomorph*

*The rounded
endomorph*

*The muscular
mesomorph*

The extent to which you can benefit from brisk, regular exercise is in part determined by your body type. You will gain more from a form of exercise that is suited to your body type than one that is not (see Section II). For example, a mesomorph is more likely to gain muscle – or gain it more quickly – than the other two types, while an ectomorph lays down fat deposits more slowly than an endomorph.

However, no matter what your genetic body type, all of us can improve and maintain our general fitness, even if some of us find it easier than others.

The amount of exercise you can do is limited by two basic biological factors:

1 How fast the cardiovascular system can deliver oxygen to the muscles

2 How effectively the muscles can extract that oxygen, thus freeing it to circulate around the body

Regular exercise can improve the efficiency of the cardiovascular system and develop the muscular system – the more you do, the more you can do and, of course, the better you will feel for it.

In general, fitness experts classify the muscles of the human body into two types: fast-twitch and slow-twitch (see pp 21–22). Endurance athletes and long-distance runners are born with 60–70% slow-twitch muscles, which are then developed through training. Sprinters are born with 60–70% fast-twitch muscles, which are also developed through training. These basic genetic types cannot be modified very much through exercise. The exercise you prefer and are best at will indicate your predominant muscle type. If you enjoy squash more than long-distance running, for example, it may be that your genetic inheritance is fast-twitch muscle.

THE BODY SYSTEMS

The systems of the body are all invigorated and toned up by regular exercise. Fitness benefits the 10 systems of the body both in the short term and the long term.

THE SYSTEMS ARE:

- The **nervous system** – the brain, spinal cord and nerves, the eyes and the ears
- The **endocrine system** – the hormone glands, which regulate many of the body's functions
- The **circulatory system** – including the heart, veins, arteries and the blood that is pumped around the body by those means
- The **digestive system** – principally the mouth, teeth, gullet, stomach, intestines and liver
- The **skeletal system** – the bones
- The **skin** – the largest single organ of the body
- The **respiratory system** – principally the lungs
- The **muscular system** – all the muscles of the body
- The **reproductive system** – including the sex glands
- The **urinary system** – the kidneys, bladder and urethra

While all body systems benefit from regular activity, three systems in particular are involved with fitness: the muscular, respiratory and cardiovascular systems.

BODY COMPOSITION

One of the best indicators of general fitness is body composition, which divides the body's weight into two categories:

- fat-free mass, primarily muscle
- fat

In fitness, what matters is how much of our weight is fat. This is usually expressed as 'per cent body fat'.

MEASUREMENT

Body composition can be measured by health professionals in a number of different ways:

- measurements of skin-fold thicknesses
- circumferences and bone diameters
- underwater weighing, regarded as one of the best methods

Once you know the volume of a body and its mass or weight you can calculate its density.

Sports scientists and health professionals at some fitness clubs and centres will be able to use the above methods and apply certain equations to estimate your body fat percentage. In this way they can assess more accurately the goals you need to achieve.

BODY IMAGE

Are you happy with your body? Do you present the
image to the world that you would like to? Not many of
us do! Body image is very closely related to self-esteem:
if you feel good about yourself, you are more likely to
be happy with your body image.

It is well known that exercise and good general fitness
improve a person's body image for a number of complex
and interrelated reasons. Physical activity is invigorating
and helps to fight feelings of lethargy. Muscular strength
improves rapidly with exercise, so you look better: your
shoulders no longer droop, your stomach is tighter,
calves and thighs take on definition, your buttocks
become firmer and posture improves. Feeling and
looking better than you did before increases your self-
esteem and general morale. It's an upward spiral.

Remember, though, you cannot alter your basic genetic
inheritance. Ectomorphs, by nature lean and slim, are
unlikely to develop a powerful musculature without
many hours of training under the guidance of a
professional trainer. Endomorphs are genetically
predisposed to gain weight and fat is likely to sit on the
stomach, buttocks and thighs. Mesomorphs, the most
muscular of the three body types, will possess more
stamina than either of the other two groups. But with
regular exercise, we can all attain a well-toned, healthy
figure and feel great in the process.

A significant pointer to general fitness and muscle tone
is the waist-to-hip ratio.

THE WAIST-TO-HIP RATIO

Women: your waist measurement divided by your hip measurement should be less than 0.8. For example, divide a 26≤ waist by 38 hips to give a ratio of 0.68 – which is fine.

Men: the same calculation should come to less than 1. For example, a 32< waist divided by 36 hips gives a ratio of 0.88 which, again, is fine. A 42≤ waist with a hip measurement of 41, however, gives a ratio of 1.02.

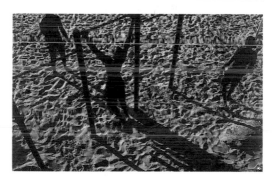

Everyone looks better as a result of regular exercise. Rightly or wrongly, body image today is more important to many of us than it has ever been before.

Body Mass Index

The Body Mass Index (BMI) ratio has superseded the
old height/weight charts as a rule of thumb indicator of
fitness. Here's how to calculate your own BMI:

1 Convert your weight to kilograms by dividing your
weight in pounds (undressed) by 2.2.

2 Convert your height in inches to metres by dividing it
by 39.4, then square it.

3 Divide (1) by (2). This is your BMI.

For example, if your weight is 65 kilograms, and height
1.68 metres, first multiply 1.68 by 1.68. That comes to
2.82. Next divide 65 by your answer (2.82). The answer,
your BMI, is 23.0.

In women a BMI of 20 to 25 means that your weight is
correct for your height, whereas a BMI of 25 to 30
indicates that you are overweight for your height. If
your BMI exceeds 30, you are very overweight. On the
other hand, a BMI of less than 15 indicates that you are
significantly underweight.

A man's BMI should be between 15 and 20. This is
because men naturally have less fat than women. The
percentage of body fat considered essential for women
is 17 per cent. A BMI less than this is a significant risk
to health. Women's higher level of fat is related to child-
bearing functions and takes into account sex-specific fat
in the breasts, hips and other tissues of the body.

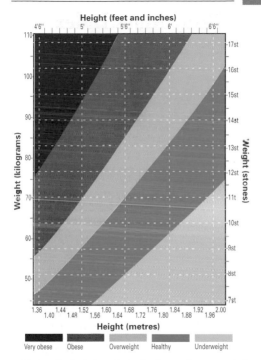

Height (feet and inches)

Weight (kilograms)

Weight (stones)

Height (metres)

| Very obese | Obese | Overweight | Healthy | Underweight |

Plot your height and weight on this chart to determine whether you are healthy, underweight or overweight.

Body metabolism

'Metabolism' is the term used to describe all of the chemical processes that occur in the body. It is controlled, in the main, by different hormones, such as adrenaline, thyroid hormones and corticosteroid hormones. The basal metabolic rate is the amount of energy needed by the body for it to function at rest, that is, for example, to maintain the heart and breathing rates and body temperature.

It is known that the body's metabolism speeds up as a result of exercise (stress and fear can also have this effect). All the systems of the body become more effective and efficient through regular, sustained activity. This means that the heart pumps oxygenated blood around the body more swiftly and more efficiently. The muscles of the body work better. When the body is tired or affected by ill health, the metabolic rate drops.

The metabolic rate is determined by the number of calories that you burn per day. There is some variation between individuals but not so great a variation as has been supposed.

Lean, underweight people are believed to have a very high metabolic rate, but the truth is that their system is actually less efficient at storing energy in the body than that of fatter individuals.

Overweight people often maintain or believe that they have a low metabolic rate – in fact they have a higher than normal metabolic rate. The reason for this is that because they have more body tissue than slimmer individuals, more energy is therefore required in order to maintain that tissue. The amount of energy used, however, is less overall because fat tissue is less metabolically active.

In order to increase the metabolic rate, therefore, you should try to increase lean muscle mass, in other words, to increase muscular fitness.

Other ways of increasing the metabolic rate include eating more in the morning and less in the evening, eating more carbohydrates and taking brisk exercise, ideally in the morning, as this will help to raise your metabolic rate for the rest of the day. Exercise lifts the metabolic rate while you are doing it, but the rate does not drop like a stone when you stop. What happens is that the metabolic rate drops gradually. For this reason, general fitness is greatly aided by, for example, two brisk walks a day – one in the morning and one in the early evening, rather than just one burst of extremely vigorous exercise once or twice a week.

It is always a good idea to avoid eating late at night, because it is then that excess energy will be stored most readily as fat.

The basal metabolic rate is measured in joules per square metre of body surface per hour. It can be tested properly only in a metabolic unit in a hospital under controlled conditions. Metabolic rate testing in certain health centres is not likely to be helpful.

Muscular fitness

In order to be fit, you need to develop your muscular fitness. We are not talking here about weight training or body building, which may develop muscular fitness at a cost to the other components of fitness.

The major muscles of the body (see diagram) all have their part to play in you becoming fit and maintaining that fitness.

There are three major types of muscle:

1 Voluntary muscles that allow you to move your limbs. There are two types: fast-twitch for bursts of energy, and slow-twitch for efficient oxygen use

2 Involuntary muscles that line the blood vessels, stomach, gastrointestinal tract and other internal organs. These smooth muscles control body functions, such as breathing and digestion, over which we have no conscious control

3 The muscles of the heart (the cardiac muscles)

Muscles are made up of overlapping bundles of fibres, which are connected to the brain by a set of nerves. These nerves carry electrical messages that tell the muscle when to contract and by how much. The result is a sliding action that causes the muscle to bulge and shorten, using up enormous amounts of energy. Regular action keeps the muscle fit and healthy and able to respond to the demands made upon it.

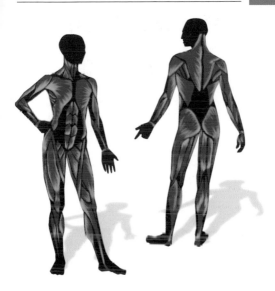

The main muscle groups of the body. Males and females have the same muscle anatomy but the male body has a significantly greater muscle mass.

Muscle accounts for some 40 per cent of our body weight and both cardiac and voluntary muscles deteriorate if they are not worked briskly and regularly.

These muscles lose strength and bulk and they gradually shrink. Most people become less muscular as they grow older, but this happens not so much as a consequence of old age but as a result of under-use.

People who are unfit start to find that they no longer have the strength or grip that they used to have: lifting a heavy box becomes difficult, gardening is more demanding than it used to be. They may experience odd aches and pains as the muscles protest against any unexpected effort. These aches and pains are not warning signs to stop what you are doing, but warning signs that the muscles have become weak and need more physical activity.

WHILE IN THE SHOWER OR BATH

Flex your shoulder muscles, lift your right arm up over your right shoulder and touch first your right shoulder blade and then your left shoulder blade. Now do the same with your left arm, touching left shoulder blade first.

Making sure you are secure and won't slip, raise your right knee up to your chin, feel your leg muscles stretch, then slowly release. Now do the same with your left knee.

Stretch and draw a circle with your left foot.

Stretch and draw a circle with your right foot.

If your legs ache when you try to walk up four or five flights of stairs, it is because the muscles of the thighs and calves have lost their ability to meet all the demands you are making upon them. In an unfit person, the cardiac muscle of the heart is also unable to pump sufficient freshly oxygenated blood around the body quickly enough to reach the struggling muscles. The result is that the muscles are not performing as well as they do in a fit person, whose muscle metabolism has its full capacity to take up oxygen from the blood and convert it into the energy needed for mechanical work.

Fortunately, the voluntary muscles respond rapidly to exercise. After only a few weeks' regular activity, these muscles will start to increase in bulk, stamina and strength. This will correspond with an increase in weight, although overall body measurements will decrease. The reason for this is that muscle is denser than fat (one pound of muscle takes the space of one third of a pound of fat).

FAST- AND SLOW-TWITCH MUSCLES

The fast- and slow-twitch muscle fibres are so called because they twitch either quickly or relatively slowly in response to the type of motor nerve that activates them. It is usually the case that the more fast-twitch fibres you have the better you can undertake explosive bursts of activity, for example, sprinting or playing squash. The more slow-twitch fibres you have, the better your capacity for forms of exercise that require endurance, such as walking, swimming and cycling.

WHILE STANDING IN A QUEUE

Flex and release the shoulder muscles of your left shoulder and then your right shoulder.

Flex and release the muscles of your left hand and then your right hand.

Hold in tightly your abdominal muscles, now release. Do this several times.

Clench and release the muscles of the buttocks – no one will know what you are doing!

Stretch and release the muscles of your left leg, and now do the same with your right leg.

Provided that you do not feel too conspicuous, stretch and describe a circle with your right foot. Now repeat with your left foot.

Fast-twitch muscles are essentially anaerobic, that is, they use fuel from the body's stores without using oxygen supplies.

Slow-twitch muscle fibres are aerobic, which means that they depend on burning glucose with oxygen from the body to release energy. Slow-twitch muscle fibre is less quick to tire.

For optimum fitness you need to enjoy several types of activity, both aerobic and anaerobic, so that both types of muscle fibre are exercised to the full. You will not be able to alter the proportion of slow-twitch fibres or fast-

Aerobic exercises result in an increase of oxygen to the muscles and organs of the body.

Aerobic = with oxygen

Examples include: jogging, running, swimming, rowing, cycling, brisk walking.

twitch fibres, but you will be able to increase their size and influence their efficiency.

You will see in Section II the many different choices available to you for keeping fit. All of the activities described use some of the muscle groups. Swimming, for example, uses most of the muscle groups. However, you can to an extent invigorate your muscles and maintain muscle tone without engaging in any of these activities, by stretching and flexing different muscles whenever you have ample time and privacy, even when you are sitting watching television, having a bath or waiting for a bus.

Anaerobic exercises require little or no oxygen. Short bursts of energy are expended.

Anaerobic = without oxygen

Examples include: sprinting, squash, weightlifting.

Respiratory fitness

We cannot live without oxygen. Activities such as lifting, running and playing golf, for example, all require energy. Energy comes from the fuel we take into the bloodstream when we digest our food. To release its energy the fuel must be combined with oxygen.

Breathing is controlled automatically by the brain (though it can also be controlled consciously if required). Nerve stimulation causes the diaphragm to contract and flatten. This increases the volume in the chest cavity and so reduces the pressure inside the chest cavity compared with outside. Air flows in from the outside, down this pressure gradient: this is inspiration. At the end of inspiration, the diaphragm relaxes and air flows out passively. Only during moderate- to high-intensity exercise do the chest muscles contribute to forcing air out of the lungs more rapidly.

Our breathing (respiratory) rate depends on how much oxygen the body needs at any one time. The normal breathing rate for an adult at rest is between 12 and 14 times a minute, although this can increase to as much as 80 times a minute when the body needs more oxygen, such as during any physical exertion. Children breathe faster than adults because they are smaller.

'GOOD' AND 'BAD' BREATHING

Most people use only a part of their lung capacity when they breathe. An average man can hold up to about 6

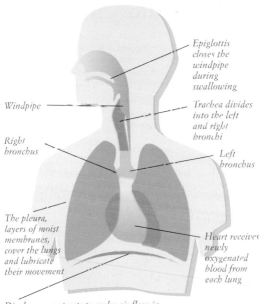

Epiglottis closes the windpipe during swallowing

Windpipe

Trachea divides into the left and right bronchi

Right bronchus

Left bronchus

The pleura, layers of moist membranes, cover the lungs and lubricate their movement

Heart receives newly oxygenated blood from each lung

Diaphragm contracts to make air flow in to the lungs. When the diaphragm muscles relax, air flows out of the lungs

The lungs are protected in the chest cavity by the ribs, spine, breastbone and respiratory muscles.

litres (10½ pints) and a woman about 4.5 litres (8 pints) of air. The lungs are divided into three sections:

- top (clavicular)
- middle (thoracic)
- bottom (abdominal)

Many people breathe using only the top section of their lungs, drawing in quick 'gasps' of breath. This chest breathing should only be used when the body is responding to a stressful situation, not as the main method of breathing. If it does become the norm, it can cause overbreathing (hyperventilation, see below).

> **In...** The diaphragm moves down, expanding the lungs. Air is drawn in through the nostrils, down the trachea and into the lungs.
>
> **... and out** The diaphragm relaxes, the lungs reduce in volume and air is expelled up through the trachea and out through the nose.

Abdominal/diaphragmatic breathing is a better way to breathe because the lungs expand more fully. This means that the body takes in more oxygen and there is also a decrease in the levels of carbon dioxide, one of the products of metabolism, a build-up of which can lead to fatigue and anxiety.

Learning to breathe deeply and slowly from the abdomen is not only good for your physical health, it is good for your mental health too. It is possible to control the rate and depth of breathing and so relax both your body and mind. The technique can be useful as a way of relieving stress and in childbirth it can help to control the painful contractions of labour.

ABDOMINAL BREATHING EXERCISE

- Sit cross-legged on the floor.

- Put your hands on your abdomen, just below your ribs.

- Close your mouth and breathe in slowly through your nose. As you do so, allow your abdomen to rise.

- Hold your breath for a few moments before slowly exhaling as much air as you can, again through your nose. As you do so, feel your abdomen fall.

- Repeat for about 5–15 minutes every day.

INCREASING RESPIRATORY FITNESS

Aerobic exercise or training is any form of exercise that makes you a little breathless (but not so seriously that you cannot continue with the activity) and forces you to breathe harder. This improves the efficiency of the delivery of oxygen around the body and also improves the energy-producing potential of the muscles. In health terms, the benefits are enormous and include fat loss, reduced likelihood of infection through the strengthening of the immune system, an improved sense of well-being and vitality in the short term, improved quality of life generally and a potential increase in life expectancy in the long term.

The aerobic system of the body is best trained by continuous and sustained exercise just below your maximum ability.

THE EFFECT OF STRESS

When we are under stress, feel frightened, anxious, very emotional or angry, the body's 'fight or flight' response is triggered. Breathing takes place in the top part of the lungs only, becoming rapid and shallow and causing a drop in the carbon dioxide levels in the blood. This leads to tiredness and anxiety and creates tension in the neck, shoulders and upper back. Breathing into a paper bag can help reduce the loss of carbon dioxide.

SMOKING

Most damaging of all to respiratory fitness is taking in smoke and tar from cigarettes, cigars and pipes. The changes in the lungs of smokers and passive smokers take place progressively and insidiously. The elasticity of the lungs, and resulting difficulty in breathing, is the first sign of deterioration. Tar, together with other substances in cigarette smoke, damages the tiny hairs in the lungs called cilia. These hairs keep the lungs clean, sweeping germs and dirt up and out of the lungs. Once the hairs are tarred up, they can no longer perform this vital respiratory function. Even one cigarette can paralyse cilia and so potentially harmful particles remain in the lungs and upper airways longer than they should. This is why smokers are especially prone to chest infections. Smoking tobacco is also responsible for increasing the likelihood of:

- a rise in blood pressure
- an increase in pulse rate
- irregular heartbeat
- reduced efficiency of the red blood cells, which are responsible for carrying oxygen around the body
- bronchitis (chronic obstruction of the airways to the lungs, which causes extreme difficulty in breathing)
- cancer of the lungs (and many other cancers)
- emphysema (the air sacs of the lungs become grossly enlarged and are eventually destroyed, making it increasingly difficult to breathe)
- arteriosclerosis (hardening of the arteries)
- atherosclerosis (narrowing of the arteries due to deposits of fat in their walls)
- angina (chest pain on exertion)
- heart attack (severe chest pain and often death)
- gangrene (death of skin and muscle, particularly in the limbs, sometimes necessitating amputation)
- stroke

The good news is that you benefit immediately from the moment you stop smoking. Call Smoker's Quitline on 0171–487 3000 for help and advice.

Cardiovascular fitness

The heart is the principal organ of the body's circulation system, known as the cardiovascular system. The circulation of the blood around the body can be described as a transport system carrying fuel and oxygen to all the cells. It is driven by a pump, the heart muscle (see diagram opposite).

The heart possesses tremendous force. You can feel the jet of blood being pumped into your arteries by placing your finger lightly on the inside of your wrist below your thumb. You will find that the heart beats about 70 times a minute. Each beat pumps out a cupful of blood.

Like any other muscle, the heart relies upon a constant supply of oxygen to maintain sustained activity. The difference between the heart and other muscles of the body is that for life to be sustained, the heart must keep working all the time.

THE IMPORTANCE OF CARDIOVASCULAR FITNESS

Cardiovascular fitness is vital in preventing diseases of the heart and arteries, caused mainly by the accumulation of a waxy substance, atheroma, on the walls of the arteries. When the coronary arteries, which supply blood to the heart, are narrowed and blocked as a result of atheroma, this becomes life threatening.

Aerobic exercise is the best way of reducing the body's

tendency to form atheroma, unless you smoke. If you are a smoker, the most important step you can take for your health is to stop smoking – then you should concentrate on increasing your aerobic exercise.

YOUR PULSE RATE

When you start to exercise, your heart quickly needs to pump more blood around the body. As you become fitter your resting pulse decreases. This improvement in heart function can be measured by taking your pulse

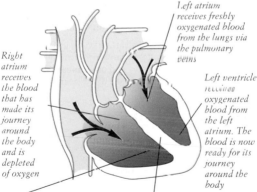

Left atrium receives freshly oxygenated blood from the lungs via the pulmonary veins

Right atrium receives the blood that has made its journey around the body and is depleted of oxygen

Left ventricle receives oxygenated blood from the left atrium. The blood is now ready for its journey around the body

Right ventricle pumps the oxygen-depleted blood through the pulmonary arteries to the lungs to pick up oxygen

Septum divides the heart into two and stops the de-oxygenated blood mixing with oxygenated blood

rate. A normal non-smoker has a pulse rate of about 65 to 70 beats a minute (a smoker's is usually about 5 to 10 beats higher).

As your aerobic fitness increases and improves, your resting pulse rate falls to about 60 beats a minute or even lower. International athletes may have resting pulse rates of 40 or less. Take your resting pulse rate in the morning, when you first wake up.

Your resting pulse rate will fall with your increased fitness and so will the rate to which it rises during moderate exercise. For example, an unfit person may have a pulse rate of 130 beats per minute when climbing a flight of stairs, whereas a fit colleague may have a rate of only 90 beats per minute. The unfit person's heart has to work much harder to achieve the same activity than the fit person's heart. In a fit person, the amount of blood the heart pumps at each beat is greater than that in the unfit person: the heart is more efficient and therefore likely to function better.

The smoker, whose heart is forced to beat up to 10 beats more per minute than the non-smoker, is clearly at a significant disadvantage when it comes to becoming fit and maintaining fitness.

YOUR BLOOD PRESSURE

Blood pressure is particularly significant as it can be used as a predictor of health.

It rises during any form of physical exertion and in

response to stress. It may even be permanently raised during periods of rest. High blood pressure (hypertension) is dangerous and can be life threatening as it damages blood vessels and can lead to stroke, heart failure and many other ailments. The heart must work harder to pump blood around the body as the arteries have become constricted

MEASURING BLOOD PRESSURE

Blood pressure is measured by reading the peak or systolic pressure in the system and the lowest or diastolic pressure that is reached in the pause between heartbeats. Your systolic pressure should be below 140 and your diastolic pressure below 90. You will find that both figures decrease as your general fitness increases.

Regular and sustained exercise reduces the resistance to blood flow caused by constricted arteries. As a result there is a fall in blood pressure.

The more tired you are, the less efficient your heart is and the more beats per minute are required to pump sufficient blood around your body. The heart must work harder. Cardiovascular fitness, achieved through regular and sustained exercise, will give you more energy. However tired you may feel, remember that you are giving your heart the boost it urgently needs when you embark on a regular exercise programme.

Diet and fitness

For reaching and maintaining optimum health and fitness, good nutrition is an essential and integral part of any exercise regime. Our bodies are nourished by the food we eat, by the liquid we drink and by the oxygen in the air we breathe. Healthy muscles depend not only on exercise but on the fuel we provide. In the same way, the heart muscle and the circulatory system depend on a healthy and varied diet.

WHAT ARE THE ELEMENTS OF GOOD DIET?

These are:

- What we eat
- When we eat
- How often we eat
- How much we eat

WHAT WE EAT

Food provides us with the fuel that we need, both for energy and repair of the body cells, to maintain life, health and fitness. The fuel that we need falls into three groups: carbohydrates, protein and fats.

Carbohydrates These provide the body with its chief source of energy. There are two categories of carbohydrates:

1 complex – we should eat more of these

2 refined – we should eat less of these

The body converts carbohydrates into glucose and glycogen in order to fuel the muscles, the nervous system and the brain. The best sources of carbohydrates are whole grains, which are to be found in wholemeal bread, pulses (beans and lentils), brown rice and wholemeal pasta. The calories from these carbohydrates burn the fastest of all and are not readily converted into body fat. Good carbohydrates also come from the natural sugars of some vegetables and fruit.

The body makes its own sugar from the healthy food that we eat. We do not need to eat any refined sugar at all. Sugar is refined from sugar cane and sugar beet and contains no fibre, no vitamins and no minerals. In addition, it is largely responsible for dental decay and obesity, and is a significant factor in heart disease and the formation of atheroma.

COMPLEX CARBOHYDRATES

- **found:** in the starch and plant cell wall materials (known as dietary fibre) in foods of plant origin

- **examples:** wheat, beans, potatoes and all fruits and vegetables

- **advantages:** slow conversion into glucose which is gradually released into the bloodstream to provide a source of long-term energy

REFINED CARBOHYDRATES

- **what are they?:** generally, high-calorie carbohydrates that have been processed or refined,
i.e. all the health-giving nutrients have been
extracted

- **examples:** refined white sugar and flour

- **disadvantages:** quickly absorbed into the
bloodstream and provide instant bursts of
energy, followed by a corresponding sense of
fatigue. Refined carbohydrates upset our natural
blood sugar levels and cannot provide the
gradual release of energy and nutrients that are
supplied by whole carbohydrates

We now consume in one fortnight the amount of sugar
that would have lasted for one entire year 200 years ago.

Protein This is essential for building new body tissue and
supplying essential amino acids, the small units of protein
that repair old cell tissue. Protein helps to build and
maintain bone and muscle and is vital to the production
of hormones and enzymes.

Protein comes in the form of meat, eggs, fish and milk.
Bread and cereals make up about one quarter of the
protein supply in the average diet: wheat, for example,
has a 10 per cent protein content.

We need only 70 grams ($2\frac{1}{2}$ ounces) of protein a day for optimum health. Any excess protein is stored in the body as fat. Many of us consume twice the amount of protein that we need. The problem with most sources of protein is that they come from animal produce and contain saturated fats which raise the blood cholesterol levels and contribute to heart disease.

Fats These are an important source of energy and help to protect the body by maintaining organs, cell structure and body temperature. They carry the fat-soluble vitamins A, D, E and K into and around the body. Some fatty acids are maufactured in the body, but others known as 'essential fatty acids' must be gained from the food we eat as we cannot produce them ourselves.

There are two types of fat: saturated fats (or saturates) and unsaturated fats (or unsaturates). The unsaturated group includes two types, polyunsaturated fats and monounsaturated fats.

THE RIGHT BALANCE

For optimum fitness we need a good balance of carbohydrate, protein and fats. In order to achieve this, all we need to do is to eat from the four main food groups each day.

The four food groups are:

1 Protein in the form of meat, poultry and fish

2 Smaller amounts of protein and calcium from dairy products such as eggs, cheese, milk and milk products

You can improve your health not only by exercising regularly but by eating some of these foods every day and avoiding junk foods. Give your body only the very best of fresh, healthy foods.

3 Protein from vegetable sources such as nuts, peas, beans, lentils, soya and pulses

4 Carbohydrate and fibre from pulses and grains (and to a much lesser extent from fruit and fresh vegetables) in the form of barley and bran, for example

To get enough fibre, you should eat one of the following at least once a day: whole-wheat cereal, wholemeal bread, wholemeal pasta, wholemeal savoury biscuits.

Precisely how much you need from each group depends on factors such as your sex, age, weight and how much energy is expended.

SATURATED FATS

- **found:** in foods of animal origin
- **examples:** dairy products, such as butter, cheese and cream, and eggs and meat
- **disadvantages:** saturated fats increase blood cholesterol levels, which in turn increase the risk of heart disease

WHEN WE EAT

In order to make the best use of the food it receives, the body needs to be stoked up in the morning with fuel, just like a fire. Eating soon after you wake raises the metabolic rate and provides you with the energy you need for the rest of the day.

'Breakfast like a king, lunch like a prince and dine like a pauper' is excellent advice for fitness and health.

If you eat large meals late in the evening, much of your intake will be converted to fat because you are not using it up in the form of energy.

HOW OFTEN WE EAT

Many of us are compelled by our lifestyles to eat perhaps only twice a day. The ideal, however, for optimum fitness and health is to eat six small meals a day. At least try to eat breakfast, lunch and supper. When you are hungry between meals, go for a healthy snack rather than chocolate or crisps.

UNSATURATED FATS

- **found**: in foods of plant origin and are predominantly polyunsaturated

- **examples**: vegetable oils which are high in polyunsaturates and monounsaturates, such as sunflower, corn, rapeseed, soya, olive, sesame, hazelnut and walnut oils. Also found in wholegrain cereals and oily fish, e.g. sardines and mackerel

- **advantages**: unsaturated fats do not cause an increase in cholesterol levels and are, therefore, better for us in reducing the risk of heart disease

HOW MUCH WE EAT

It is important to listen to your body and eat when you are hungry. There is no point in eating a big dinner if you are not particularly hungry. Just eat some fruit instead.

Nearly half the population is now considered to be

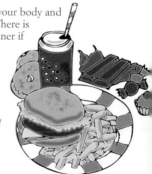

For good general health, avoid these foods: iced buns, fizzy drinks, chocolate, sweets and fatty take-away foods, especially chips.

overweight. We are all eating too much refined sugar, chocolate, crisps and junk food, all of which provide some nutrition but a lot of calories.

The serious medical issues associated with being overweight and obese may seem remote if you are only a few pounds overweight and in your twenties. But as you age, it becomes harder to lose weight and only too easy to gain it. You may be less active and your metabolism will have slowed down. So try to establish healthy eating habits now and help yourself keep to a healthy weight.

THE WARNING SIGNS
OF BEING OVERWEIGHT

- feeling tired
- shortness of breath
- fluid retention
- aches and pains
- swelling of the joints, especially at the hip and knee
- back problems
- foot problems, such as collapsed arches and bunions
- indigestion
- constipation

Fitness in children

The habits acquired in childhood are important in adult life. If you become used to walking and cycling as a child and to eating healthily and regularly, you have a better chance of maintaining these habits in adult life than if you had never experienced them as a child.

Children need fresh air and exercise, even more than adults, in order for their muscles to develop and for their bones to grow. Carbohydrate foods such as wholemeal breads and pasta provide energy for the muscles, and the protein found in dairy foods is essential for strong bones.

Many experts are concerned at fitness levels in today's children. There are a number of reasons for this:

1 Children walk far less than they used to. For example, many children are driven rather than walk to school

2 Children play outdoors less than they used to. Parents are more concerned these days to know where their children are and what they are doing. Children spend several hours a week in sedentary activity, such as watching television and playing with computers

3 Children's diets comprise too much fast food, fried food, chocolate, crisps, sweets, fizzy drinks and convenience foods

4 Girls, especially, are concerned with losing weight. Forty per cent of thin girls diet constantly, despite the

fact there is no need to and despite the fact their bodies are not being properly nourished. Exaggerated ideals of slenderness have led to many adolescents becoming dissatisfied with their body shape and complaining about bulging hips, fat tums, big bottoms and wobbly thighs.

It is essential to instil healthy exercise and dietary habits in children at as young an age as possible. Never let your children go out of the house without first eating breakfast. Make sure that they have a healthy lunch, either as a packed lunch or lunch at school.

Children, and especially adolescents, need a lot of fuel and they are likely to want snacks between meals. Offer them any of these: fruit, vegetables, healthy nut bars, a wholemeal sandwich with cheese or tuna and salad.

Exercise in the sunlight is essential for the formation of healthy young bones.

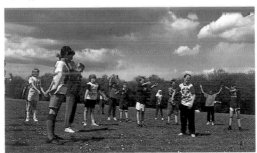

Explain to them what chocolate and crisps (fat) and sweets (refined sugar) are doing to their bodies, that there is no really healthy nutrition in these foods and that when they eat them, their bodies receive an artificial boost of energy that will be followed by a corresponding drop, so the 'high' is short-lived.

Children under the age of two should only be given full-fat products. From the age of five onwards reduced-fat products can be introduced into their diets, but only if they are good eaters. Meat eaters, for example, will have less need for full-fat products than vegetarian eaters. But children of all ages, especially girls, should be given full-fat milk.

Toddlers can learn to swim even before they learn to walk and this should be encouraged. Section II contains many options for becoming fit, and children should be encouraged to pick one or two for themselves to do at the weekend. During the school week, encourage your child to take part in physical activities, especially competitive games.

Many children are loath to go for a walk for the pleasure of it, but the walk can be combined with some interesting pursuit or goal to persuade the child to walk. For example, walk to the tennis court, football pitch or cricket field. Walk to the swimming baths. Walk to the fair or the circus or the shops. Buy your child a kite, so that you both have a reason to go out walking. Try to incorporate walking into your and your children's lifestyle, both for their health and your own.

FITNESS PRESENTS FOR KIDS

Make fitness fun by choosing Christmas and birthday presents that involve some kind of physical activity and lead them away from sedentary pastimes. For example:

- climbing frame
- skipping rope
- bicycle
- table tennis table
- mini football table
- mini snooker table
- rollerblades or ice skates
- football
- frisbee
- boules (both for beach and garden)
- croquet set for the family
- toboggan/sledge
- kite
- pedometer to monitor the distance that they walk
- rope ladder to attach to a tree in the garden

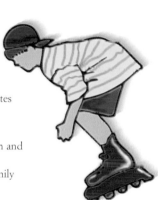

Children suffer more heat gain in extreme heat than adults, and greater heat loss in cold weather than adults. They should have extra layers of clothing to put on after physical activity, and be encouraged to drink water (not carbonated drinks) in order to replace lost fluid.

Fitness in pregnancy

Fitness during pregnancy, and in the period before conception when you are trying to become pregnant, focuses equally on physical activity and nutrition, both for you and for your growing baby, together with some other factors. These are the principal concerns of the pregnant woman:

- Sleep
- Nutrition
- Exercise and fresh air
- Avoiding smoky atmospheres (and giving up smoking if you have not already done so)
- Cutting out or cutting down on alcohol

SLEEP

The amount of sleep you get is almost as important as when you sleep. You will benefit most by getting up at the same time each morning and going to bed at roughly the same time each evening. Don't be surprised to find that you need much more sleep than usual.

Avoid lying and sleeping on your back as this impedes your blood circulation and may contribute to you feeling cold and your ankles and wrists swelling.

Take an afternoon nap whenever the opportunity arises. If you are working full-time, try to pace yourself as sensibly as possible. Make use of your lunch hour to rest rather than whizzing around the shops. Can you avoid the rush hour by leaving half an hour earlier each day?

NUTRITION

All you need to remember is to eat from the four main food groups, described on pp 37–38, each day and to eat at least three times a day, preferably more often.

- Take your lightest meal in the evening.
- For optimum health, cut out coffee, alcohol, sugar, cakes, biscuits, sweets and highly processed foods that contain a lot of additives and preservatives.
- Avoid all soft and blue-veined cheeses and products that contain unpasteurized milk.
- You should avoid lightly cooked or raw eggs.
- You may find that you want to eat extra milk, cheese and yoghurt in response to the growing baby's demands for calcium. If so, add grated cheese to pasta dishes and to salads and drink more milk.
- To avoid constipation, a common problem during pregnancy, eat lots of foods containing fibre, such as whole-wheat cereals, wholemeal breads and wholemeal pasta.
- Eat foods rich in iron, such as lean red meat, fish, eggs and green-leaf vegetables, such as spinach.
- Folic acid is important, especially in the three months before and after conception. Look for bread and cereals with added folic acid, eat green-leaf vegetables or take 400 mcg folic acid supplement every day.

EXERCISE AND FRESH AIR

Daily exercise in fresh air and sunlight is especially important for pregnant women. Performing exercises in the privacy of your bedroom is good for you, but doing the same exercises outdoors on a sunny day or taking a good long walk each day will double the benefit.

Sunlight is essential for the formation of vitamin D and your lungs benefit by breathing in fresh air rather than the stale air of an office or home.

Avoid more hazardous sports during pregnancy, such as squash, riding, skiing, water-skiing and windsurfing, but there are plenty of other physical activities and sports that are perfectly safe (see Section II).

Swimming is without doubt the best possible exercise for the pregnant woman. You are weightless in the water and you can therefore increase your suppleness and stamina without making an enormous effort. Many sports and leisure centres run aquanatal classes, which combine exercises in the water and by the poolside.

Walking in flat, supporting shoes is very beneficial. If you walk briskly every day for at least 15 minutes, you improve your cardiovascular and respiratory fitness, and also your general muscular fitness, which will stand you in good stead for labour.

It is important to be supple and flexible as well as powerful for labour. You may find that yoga, t'ai chi and the Alexander Technique will all contribute to suppleness, but don't overdo it. Your joints and ligaments become softer during pregnancy in preparation for birth, making you more flexible than normal.

It is especially important when you are pregnant to listen to what your body is telling you, and to do the warm-up and cool-down exercises described on pp 68–75.

Check with your doctor that it is safe to embark on any exercise programme. Don't attempt to do anything that you would have found strenuous even before you were pregnant.

If you experience any of the following, stop exercising immediately and rest:

- breathlessness
- dizziness
- pain or feeling of tightness in the abdominal area, chest, arms, back or joints
- any sort of headache
- unusual fatigue or feeling of inertia

If any of the symptoms persist for more than 5 to 10 minutes, consult your doctor.

CAUTION

Don't overdo things: your body is already working hard every minute of the day as it copes with the demands of your growing baby.

EXERCISES

Ten to 15 minutes a day of a varied programme of exercises is sufficient to keep you in shape. Choose from any of the following, which you will find in Section II, but do not devote an entire session to any one particular exercise: warm-ups, cool-downs, aquaerobics, yoga, aerobics, step exercises, stretch and tone exercises.

Each exercise is designed to achieve one or more of the different types of fitness that you need in pregnancy and labour:

- deep even breathing
- improved muscle tone
- the ability to relax
- good posture, which will prevent the backache typical in pregnancy
- good circulation, which will make sure that you and your baby receive sufficient oxygen and prevent oedema (swelling at wrists and ankles)

CONTROLLING YOUR BREATHING

It is most important to become aware of your breathing during pregnancy so that you are ready for labour.

Place a pillow on the floor to support your head and lie down. Make a conscious effort to relax, breathing moderately and slowly to avoid dizziness. Place your hands on either side of your body, where you can feel your lower ribs and breathe in and out, feeling your body rise and fall as you breathe first in, then out.

When you breathe in, breathe in through your nose, and then breathe out through your mouth, blowing lightly at the same time.

Continue with this moderate and slow breathing exercise, which is also, incidentally, a wonderful method of relaxation. As you breathe in, feel your abdominal area rise, then as you breathe out contract your abdominal muscles and use this action to force the air out of your mouth.

When you are in labour, regular even breathing helps to ensure that both you and your baby receive sufficient oxygen. It may also help to take the edge off the pain. During labour you will need to push as you breathe out. Just before you are about to deliver, you will be asked not to push, despite an almost overwhelming urge to do exactly that, while either midwife or doctor checks that the umbilical cord is safely positioned for the baby to be born. The way to do this is to breathe out or blow softly or pant, and this is something you can practise during pregnancy. It is very important that you do not push when you are instructed not to otherwise the baby may be expelled too forcibly.

You will probably be taught several other exercises at your antenatal classes, and these may include back exercises to relieve backache, and pelvis and pelvic floor exercises which are designed to strengthen your pelvic muscles.

In order to maintain good circulation, do some of the exercises described on pp 20–22.

Fitness in later life

As we get older, our muscles gradually weaken, joints stiffen, bones become more brittle, arteries harden and lung capacity is reduced. Hence the mysterious aches and pains, wrenched muscles after unaccustomed exercise, breathlessness and fatigue that won't disappear with a good night's sleep.

The good news is that some regular exercise every day will build up and maintain muscle strength and tone, improve your circulation and lung capacity, and keep your joints mobile. Weight-bearing exercise, such as walking, strengthens the bones and is particularly good

Swimming is the best all-round exercise activity for working all the main muscle groups and increasing stamina and suppleness. It is never too late to learn. Many pools have over-60s sessions.

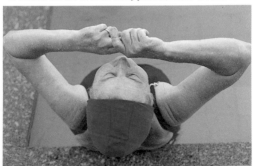

HERE'S WHAT EXERCISE CAN DO FOR YOU

- It will make you feel more energetic

- It will make you feel less anxious and stressed

- It will help you to sleep better

- It will help to keep your joints and muscles in good working order

- It will help you to lose weight and achieve or maintain a healthy weight

- It will lower your blood's cholesterol level

- It will reduce your risk of high blood pressure by up to 40 per cent

- It can reduce your risk of heart attack by over 40 per cent

- It can reduce your risk of stroke by 33 per cent

- It will reduce the risk of diabetes by 29 per cent

- It stimulates the formation of new bone to reduce your risk of a hip fracture by 60 per cent

- It can reduce your risk of breast cancer

If you exercise moderately for 30 minutes a day, you will almost halve your risk of a heart attack compared to someone who is physically inactive.

Source. Health Education Authority

for older women, who are more at risk from
osteoporosis, a condition in which the bones become
weak and brittle. Take it easy in the beginning and aim
to work up to about 20–30 minutes, five times a week.
If you are over 60, it is advisable to choose a more
gentle regime.

TYPES OF EXERCISE

All of these activites are recommended for people over
the age of 50, and many sports and leisure centres run
classes especially for this age group:

- t'ai chi and yoga, great for toning muscles and
  improving poor circulation
- rambling, walking and hiking
- games such as golf, volleyball, softball, badminton
  and bowling
- swimming, especially good as your weight is
  supported by the water and shock to tissues and
  joints is avoided
- cycling

THE GOLDEN RULES

- If you are in any doubt whatsoever about your ability
  to exercise, check with your family doctor first.
- Don't exercise after a heavy meal, if you feel unwell
  or after drinking alcohol.
- Drink a glass of water about 15 minutes before you
  start your activity.

- Always do the warm-up exercises for 10 minutes before you start.
- Stop and rest if you become seriously short of breath.
- When starting don't do more than half an hour.

WALK YOUR WAY TO FITNESS

Walking to a structured programme is one of the best ways of achieving fitness for the over-50s. Once you have completed the programme, you can then embark on the chosen activity or sport of your choice from Section II.

- Weeks 1 and 2: walk for 10 minutes, briskly, three times a week
- Weeks 3 and 4: walk for 10 minutes briskly, four times a week
- Weeks 5 and 6: walk for 10 minutes briskly, five times a week
- Weeks 7 and 8: walk for 15 minutes briskly, five times a week
- Weeks 9 and 10: walk for 20 minutes briskly, five times a week
- Week 11: walk for 25 minutes briskly, five times a week
- Week 12 and subsequent weeks: walk for 30 minutes briskly, five times a week

- Don't exercise on consecutive days until you are fit – allow a day for the body to rest and repair itself.
- When you finish, do the cool-down exercises for 10 minutes.
- Drink some more water.

ACTIVE HOBBIES

Ballroom dancing and bowls are good examples of hobbies that will increase your fitness levels. If you enjoy gardening, do as much as you can: fresh air combined with exercise is a certain way to fitness.

STEP 'N' STRETCH

If you don't feel like going out, you can exercise at home. Use the stairs as a step machine and simply walk up and walk down, walk up again and walk down again. If you don't have stairs, place a couple of telephone directories on the floor on top of one another and step on to them, step off, step on again, step off again.

Stop and raise your arms above your head. Stretch out one arm, then the other. Next, hold on to something for support and, standing on leg, stretch the other round you in a circle. Repeat with the other leg.

And now back to the step exercises. This time, walk up the stairs more briskly than you did the last time.

Once you have attained a satisfactory level of fitness, you may be surprised at how easy it is to maintain it and how much better you feel for it.

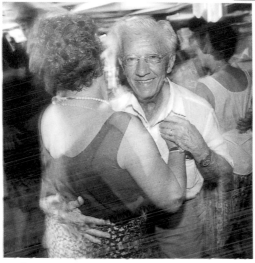

Ballroom dancing is sociable, fun and excellent for gently raising your fitness levels and improving coordination.

KEEP A DIARY

It is a good idea to note each day what physical activity you did, how long you did it for, and how you felt afterwards. This is a good way to monitor your progress. But the key is to proceed slowly and surely. Don't overdo it, or you could injure yourself.

WORKING OUT
Strength, stamina and suppleness

These are the keywords in fitness. We are aiming for all-round strength, stamina and suppleness. This means muscular, respiratory and cardiovascular strength and endurance, and muscular suppleness or flexibility.

In the following pages, you will find information about different physical activities and sports. Each of these benefits the body in different ways: some provide excellent all-round exercise (such as swimming), while others provide advantages for part but not all of the body (such as cycling). Weight training is a further example of exercise that is excellent for building strength but does little for stamina or flexibility. With activities

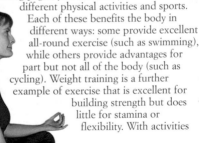

This basic yoga pose enables you to monitor and deepen your breathing, to hold your spine in the optimum position and to relax after a challenging day. Yoga develops strength, muscular endurance and suppleness all in one.

such as this, it is especially important to carry out the warm-up and cool-down exercises as they provide the body with opportunities to stretch and thus to enhance flexibility.

It is important to choose a varied exercise programme. If, for example, your favoured activity is rowing, then complement it with walking or cycling so that all parts of the body are fully exercised. As another example, if you enjoy golf, complement it with weight training at the gym. In this way, golf develops your suppleness, and training with weights enhances your power, which will in turn benefit your golf game.

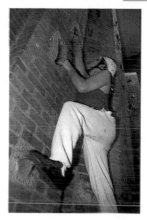

Rock climbing is a fun and ideal way to general fitness, increasing strength, flexibility, endurance and balance. Many sports centres now have indoor climbing walls on which you can practise.

Finally, reduce the risk of injury and improve your performance in your chosen exercise by warming up for 5–10 minutes with some form of continuous but relatively easy exercise, such as running on the spot. This will also help to boost your energy levels.

Cardiovascular fitness through exercise

The consequence of achieving cardiovascular fitness through exercise is that the heart will beat fewer times per minute and will adapt to pump a larger volume of blood around the body with each beat. To realize this benefit, you need to exercise energetically enough to reach your training zone – i.e. continuous activity that pushes up your heart rate to 60–90% of your maximum heart rate (the 220 minus age equation) – and then continue with the exercise for a sustained period.

YOUR TRAINING ZONE

220 minus age x 90% = ... upper limit
220 minus age x 60% = ... lower limit

First, take your resting pulse. This should ideally be done in the morning when you first get up. Simply place the index and middle fingers of your right hand on the inside of your left wrist until you feel your pulse. Using the second hand on a clock or wristwatch, count the beats you feel in 15 seconds and multiply by four. This will give you your resting pulse rate.

A normal resting pulse rate is usually around 70 to 75, but a rate of up to 90 could still be within the normal range. If you hit over 90, you should consult your doctor before indulging in any strenuous exercise.

A resting pulse rate of 60 is very good. The extra workload for the heart of someone who has 90 heartbeats per minute, compared with the person whose heart beats at 60 per minute, is substantial – 30 beats per minute's difference. In an hour this amounts to 1800 beats and in one day adds up to 43,000 extra beats. That is a lot of extra work for the heart, which could be avoided by achieving fitness.

When you are exercising, your heart rate increases as the heart works harder to pump more blood around the body. For real cardiovascular benefit you should exercise in your training zone for 20 minutes, three to five times a week. Do not push yourself beyond the top of the upper limit of your training zone, and the minimum you should aim for is the bottom of the lower limit. Regular cardiovascular exercise will, over time, result in a fall in your resting pulse rate as well as the rate to which it rises during exercise.

As your fitness increases, your heart rate will decrease as your heart becomes stronger and more efficient – it will not have to work so hard to achieve the same result.

Take your resting pulse rate first thing in the morning when you get up and before you start exercising. Take it again after exertion. How quickly your pulse rate returns to normal is a measure of your overall fitness.

Respiratory fitness through exercise

Regular and sustained exercise forces the lungs to work harder than usual. In order to do this, your body falls back on the lungs' reserve capacities and so develops them, which in turn causes the lungs to become fitter and stronger.

For exercise to be effective for the respiratory system, you need to become warm and a little out of breath. And you need to continue with the exercise at that point rather than stop and slow down to your normal respiratory rate. Breathlessness and a flushed appearance show that you are making the lungs work at a greater rate than normal.

You should not exercise to the point where you become bright red and cannot speak for breathlessness. You should always be working below your maximum ability. When walking briskly, for example, you should be able to carry on a conversation at the same time.

All forms of exercise enhance your respiratory fitness, but the endurance sports such as jogging, running, swimming and cycling do so to best effect because they provide steady and sustained exercise. Squash and boxing, in contrast, are less beneficial in that your lungs are not compelled to work at full strength for long periods. However, the combination of squash and running makes an ideal exercise programme.

Finally, try to avoid smoky atmospheres because smoke and the tar it contains are extremely damaging to all aspects of fitness.

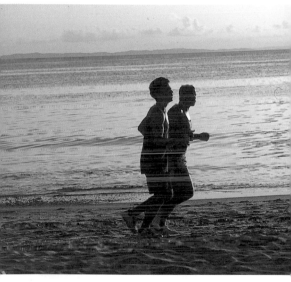

For maximum respiratory fitness, the best environment for exercise is in the fresh air, ideally by the sea. A brisk walk or a run along a beach two to three times a week will do wonders for your fitness and well-being.

Muscular fitness through exercise

It is probably your muscular fitness that you will notice the most when you first start increasing your exercise programme. You may observe that your calves have

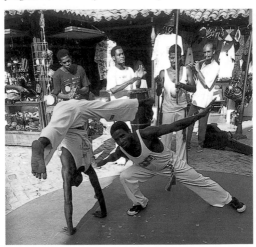

Gymnastics and martial arts enthusiasts can testify to the tremendous benefits in muscular, cardiovascular and respiratory fitness. This is optimum vitality at its most dynamic.

better definition, your posture is better, your stomach is less flabby and your bottom more taut.

Every form of exercise shown in this section will benefit your muscular fitness, some more than others and some in different ways from others. Riding, for example, will work wonders for the muscles of your thighs and calves, while canoeing or rowing will greatly benefit your shoulder and arm muscles. It is desirable to exercise all the muscle groups, and for this reason it is best to combine two or more different types of exercise.

Only one form of exercise challenges all the muscle groups and that is swimming. Many experts claim that there is no better exercise.

Remember that you can enhance your muscular tone even while watching television or queuing in the supermarket, by clenching and releasing all the muscle groups of the body in turn.

Women sometimes worry that they will become too muscular to retain a feminine appearance but this is unlikely. Women have less muscle mass than men and are therefore less likely to become muscular. This is because women do not possess the same balance of hormones as men.

You may find that although you may look slimmer and better defined as a consequence of your exercise programme, your weight has remained the same or actually increased. This is because muscle weighs three times more than fat. This is healthier.

Preparing for exercise

When you're choosing your types of exercise, look for those that combine the greatest benefits with the most enjoyment – so that you're more likely to keep them up.

THE AIM

Regular exercise will increase the effectiveness of your cardiovascular, respiratory and muscular systems (see pp 18–33). How much they improve will depend on how hard your body works when you exercise. You can check this by taking your pulse before and after exercising (see pp 60–61). Fit adults should aim to increase their heart rate to between 60 and 90% of the maximum heart rate for 20–60 minutes, three to five times a week. Regular exercise also helps in maintaining a healthy weight. Calorific expenditure (see Factfiles in Working out) will depend on many factors, such as sex, height, weight and the intensity of the particular exercise chosen. They are given as a rough guide only.

TYPE OF EXERCISE

Some of the most effective types of exercise are given in Section II. When choosing one, think about your general health, age and body type (see p 8), and practical considerations like cost, time and availability.

INTENSITY

It is important to start slowly and build up gradually.

The ideal to aim for is half an hour's brisk exercise five times a week. But you need to start with maybe only 10 to 15 minutes three times a week. If you go all out in your first session your body will become overtired and will take longer to rest and repair damaged cells – you may even pull a muscle and put yourself out of action for a week or two.

If you ever experience the warning signs of pain and severe breathlessness, you should stop.

ALL-ROUND FITNESS

Try to combine exercises that develop all the different parts of your body. Yoga, swimming, athletics and golf are all good for improving mobility as they involve bending, stretching and rotating movements.

Repeated actions such as working with weights, push-ups, squat jumps and curl-ups will build up muscle strength and stamina and help muscles to protect the joints and internal organs.

Continuous, vigorous action over an extended period of time improves the performance of the heart and lungs. Cycling, swimming, running/jogging and games such as tennis and football are all good for this.

Always check with your GP before starting any type of exercise programme and wear the correct safety wear for the activity you have chosen.

Warm-up exercises

It is important to warm up for about 5 to 10 minutes
before you start exercising to stretch the muscles and
make them more flexible and allow the body's
temperature to rise gradually. This promotes blood flow
to the working muscles for a more effective workout. In
contrast, launching into strenuous physical exercise

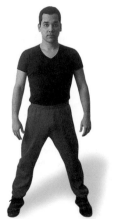
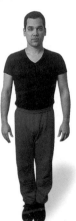

*Your basic positions for the side steps. Stand with your feet
apart, move the right foot to the right, close the left foot up to it.
Repeat, then move the left foot to the left and close the right
foot up to it.*

from a standstill presents a considerable shock to the muscles and the cardiovascular system. The lungs and the heart are forced to make huge 'leaps' in order to keep up with the demand for oxygen. An unnecessary strain is placed on these organs, which is not desirable for optimum health and fitness.

SIDE STEPS

Stand with your feet apart. Move your right leg to the right, close your left up to it. Take another sideways step with your right foot again and join up with the left. Now take one step to the left with your left foot.

Bring your right foot behind the left foot. Take a step to the left with the left foot. Now take the right foot to join the left foot and repeat the sequence five times.

Now repeat the sequence, stepping to the left this time, and repeat five times.

KNEE BENDS

Place your feet about hip distance apart and, keeping your back straight, bend your knees and lower your bottom, then stand up straight.

Repeat 10 times.

MARCHING, LOW KNEES

Raise each foot slightly from the floor and put it back again. You should bend your knees only slightly. This exercise is simply marching on the spot, but you should

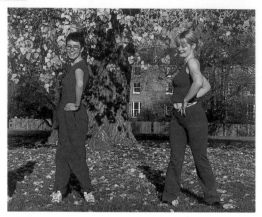

Make waist twists part of your warm-up routine. Stretch the oblique abdominal muscles by placing your hands on your waist or just above the hip, whichever is the most comfortable for you, and twist slowly from side to side.

not be lifting your feet too high because this is a low-impact exercise designed to minimize strain on your joints. Do this for about a minute.

SHOULDER CIRCLES, SHRUGS

Push your left shoulder forward slowly until you feel the muscles at the back of your shoulder stretching. Push your shoulder back this time, again until you feel the muscles at the back of it stretching.

Do each movement five times, then repeat the sequence with your right shoulder.

Now stand relaxed and shrug your shoulders up to your neck, and let them fall back again. Repeat ten times.

WAIST TWISTS

Stand with your feet slightly apart, so that they are in line with your hips. Slowly twist your upper body to the right and slowly return. Repeat five times.

Now repeat the sequence, twisting your upper body to the left and slowly returning each time.

TOUCHING YOUR TOES

Let your body fall forward from the waist in as relaxed a manner as possible. Consciously allow your neck to relax. Point your fingers towards your toes. Don't strain to touch your toes until after you have exercised and the body is thoroughly toned up.

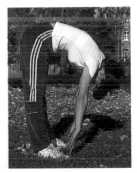

When you touch your toes, be sure that your neck is completely relaxed and allow your head to drop down towards your toes. Keep your legs straight, but don't force yourself to stretch more than is comfortable for you.

Cool-down exercises

First, drink a glass of water to replace the body fluids lost during exercise. Water is far better for you than a fizzy drink.

When you stop exercising, your body will cool down quite rapidly. One good reason for performing cool-down exercises for a short period after brisk or strenuous activity is to prevent your blood pressure from dropping too quickly. If this happens, it may cause you to feel faint.

Cool-down exercises also allow the blood flow to be maintained and oxygen to be supplied to the entire body. Have to hand a fleece, tracksuit top or a sweater. If you are exercising outdoors in winter, have with you a woollen hat, warm

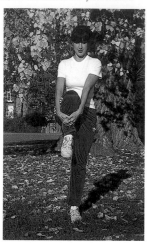

Part of your cool-down routine should include stretching tense muscles while they are still warm. Stretch out the hamstrings as shown by hugging your calf – see if your raised foot can make contact with your buttock for maximum stretch.

gloves and a scarf as well. In this way, your body cools down slowly.

LEG STRETCHES

Place your hands on your hips. Extend your left leg straight out in front of you. Now tilt the body forward and allow the back leg (the right leg) to bend at the knee. This takes some concentration to achieve as the natural tendency is to bend the forward (left) leg. It is an excellent exercise for extending the muscles of the thighs and calves.

Now repeat with the right leg forward, unbent, and the left leg behind, bent.

Feel the stretch in your hamstrings and the challenge to your hip joints.

Repeat these exercises, slowly, alternating your right and left leg for three or four minutes.

SIDE SLIDES

Stand with your feet slightly apart, wide enough so that your feet are in line with your hips. Then with your right arm hanging loosely by your right side, bend your upper body to the right so that your right hand slides down your right leg. Slowly pull your body

Some people find it easier to start in this position when doing leg stretches. This is good for the muscles of the legs and buttocks.

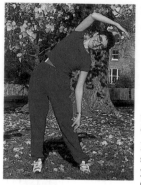

Left: Your cool-downs should include a couple of minutes of side slides to stretch the oblique abdominal muscles. Keep your body upright, and avoid head and upper body projecting forward.

up again. Repeat the exercise five times.

Now repeat the exercise, slowly, this time using your left hand to run down your left leg.

Now slowly repeat the sequences first with your right hand/leg and then your left hand/leg.

You should spend up to 10 minutes doing your cool-down exercises. It is up to you to make a selection of those that exercise each part of your body best. Choose from waist twists, side steps, knee bends, touching your toes, low marching, shoulder circles and

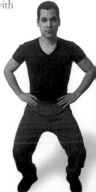

Right: When you are doing knee bends, be sure to keep your back upright and your eyes looking straight ahead. The neck and shoulders should be relaxed.

shrugs, all of which are described on pp 68–71.

Many people like to go for a leisurely walk after brisk or intense physical activity – such as squash or boxing, for example – and this makes an excellent cooling-down exercise. You should still follow your walk with about five minutes of cooling-down exercises.

Finally, don't forget to drink at least one glass of water after exercise and preferably more.

For maximum benefit hold this stretch for 30 seconds. Now stretch the other side of the body. Be sure to keep the neck and shoulders relaxed.

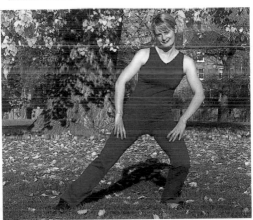

Walking

You can walk for pleasure in accordance with a structured programme or alternatively incorporate walking into normal everyday life. There are many different ways of walking: slow, brisk, fast and power-walking, all of which have beneficial effects. Walking is without doubt one of the very best all-round exercises for muscular, cardiovascular and respiratory fitness.

A brisk (about 6.4kph/4 mph) half-hour walk, five days a week will provide exercise for the heart, stomach muscles, arms and legs (without straining the joints) and is a great stress-reliever. Moreover, walking is not just an outdoor activity. Although perhaps less enjoyable, it can be done indoors. A treadmill can be used regardless of the weather and provides the same benefits to the heart, lungs and legs.

When you walk, keep your shoulders wide and relaxed, and let your arms hang loosely by your side so that they swing backward and forward naturally as you walk.

HOW MUCH DO YOU WALK?

- Do you go for a walk when you first get up in the morning?
- Do you walk to the shops?
- Have you ever thought of having a dog so that walking twice a day would have to become part of your daily routine?

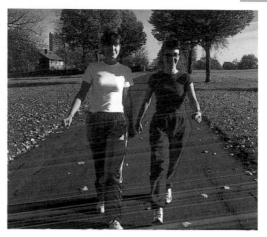

Brisk walking is an invigorating activity that is excellent for all-round fitness and appropriate for all age groups as well as for pregnant women. Aim for 30 minutes at a brisk pace each day.

- Could you walk to work?
- Could you get off the bus one or two stops before your destination and walk the rest of the way?
- When faced with a lift or escalator in shops and railway stations, think of your heart and the muscles of your body, and seize your chance for increased fitness: walk up instead.

FACTFILE

Calories burnt per minute: 3–9, depending on the rate of walking

Benefits: good cardiovascular, respiratory and muscular fitness

Works on: stamina in legs, stomach muscles, shoulders and arms

Complementary exercise: any

You need: a water bottle, supportive footwear

- Do you walk for pleasure in the park or in the country at least once a week?
- If your job is largely sedentary, are there ways in which you could make it more physically active for yourself?

You can monitor your speed of walking and the distance, as well as the calories consumed, on a treadmill. You can set the machine for walking on flat ground or for walking uphill (even better for cardiovascular, respiratory and muscular fitness).

- Do your legs ache when you climb steps? Even if it is just a short flight? That's a clear warning sign that you need to walk a lot more in order to tone up those complaining muscles.

- When you are at home, do you put things at the bottom of the stairs to take up later? Seize the opportunity and take them up now. Make several trips if necessary and revel in the easy availability of another opportunity for activity.

Walking is a suitable fitness activity for all age groups – young (get them into the walking habit early on), pregnant and elderly people. And it's free.

The Ramblers' Association (see Useful addresses) has over one hundred thousand members of all ages throughout the United Kingdom. Walks are graded in difficulty and can range from a 5-km (3-mile) walk along a river to a strenuous mountain climb.

The heel of your foot should strike the ground first, then your whole foot and you should push off for the next step on the ball of the foot. This correct style of walking is best for your spine, your feet and your propulsion.

Golf

Golf makes an excellent exercise for all age groups. You are walking in the fresh air, sometimes for several miles up and down hills, while carrying your golf clubs, and you are developing your muscular fitness and flexibility in the swing and the strike. (Leave the wheeled carrier and the buggy at the clubhouse if you want to become fit.) It needs and promotes mobility, you need to have good posture, balance, and a sense of rhythm.

Do some warm-up and stretch 'n' tone exercises before you play a round. They are particularly beneficial for your flexibility and power. Freedom in the neck muscles, particularly in the older golfer, is essential to allow the body and shoulders to turn fully while the head stays still, eyes focused on the ball.

Practise your swing at home, in a public park, or , best of all, on a public golf course (where you will be required to pay a small fee) before you join a club.

Postural control is of supreme importance in golf in the moments just before you hit the ball, and you also need good striking power. You need to be supple to have a good follow through towards the end of your stroke.

After loosening the neck muscles (see pp 82–83), try this for the shoulders:

Hold your driver in front of you, arms straight, left hand at the top of the grip and right hand down by the head of the club. Bring the club back over your head, keeping the arms straight, and then return it to the starting point. The looser and freer your shoulders are, the shorter the club you can use for this exercise.

TWIST THE CLUB

To loosen up your back, hold a club behind your back passing your arms over the club so that it is held between both elbows in the back. Now twist your body first to the left and then to the right. Ease yourself round as far as you can to loosen up the muscles in the upper body and lower back.

FACTFILE

Calories burnt per minute: 3.8–6.2

Works on: mobility, flexibility and strength in the arms, shoulders and back; is good for posture

Complementary exercises: weights, swimming

Stretch 'n' tone

Flexibility is an essential part of fitness and yet many athletes and sports players neglect this aspect of their training. Increased flexibility is believed to prevent injury and may well enhance your speed. Stiff, creaking joints mean that you need to focus on increasing your flexibility through stretch 'n' tone exercises. Start with the warm-up exercises shown on pp 68–71.

YOUR NECK AND SHOULDERS

- Lift your head up and back and stretch your neck to its full height. Slowly turn it to the right and then to the left. Dip your head and return to looking straight ahead.

- Slowly rotate your head in a clockwise and then anti-clockwise direction.

- Open out your shoulders with your elbows coming away from your waist.

- Take your shoulders back as far as

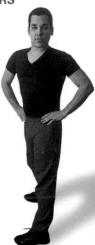

Stretch 'n' tone your oblique abdominal muscles and the muscles of your back with side stretches. To do this, place your hands on your hips or waist and stretch slowly and fully, first to one side and then the other.

FACTFILE

Calories burnt per minute: 4

Works on: flexibility in the arms, legs, shoulders, neck, back and stomach

they will go. Lift your left shoulder and relax it down again. Now lift and relax your right shoulder.

- Swing your right arm slowly in a full circular movement to free the shoulder.
- Swing your left arm in the same way.
- Raise and relax both shoulders.
- Repeat the neck exercises.
- Put your right hand over your right shoulder and touch your left shoulder blade.
- Repeat with your left hand to your right shoulder.

ABDOMINAL STRETCH

- Lie on your back on the floor, with knees bent. Extend your stomach upwards as far as you can.

Stretch the muscles of your buttocks and thighs by bringing one foot over the other thigh and at the same time raising the lower foot.

The body weight is resting on your feet and shoulders.
Your abdominal muscles are fully stretched.

SIDE STRETCH

- Stand with your feet about hip-width apart. Bend
  your upper body sideways to the right and count to
  15 – don't lean forward. Repeat to the left. This
  stretches the oblique abdominal muscles.

LOWER BACK AND HAMSTRINGS

- Sit on the floor, place your feet together and your
  legs straight out in front of you. Sit up and then
  stretch forward as far as you can towards your toes.
- With your legs slightly apart, repeat.
- Now touch your left toes with your right hand and
  then your right toes with your left hand. You should

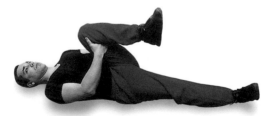

*Strengthen the muscles of your lower back, the buttocks and
your hamstrings by clasping first one thigh and bringing it up to
your chest and then the other. Bring each thigh up slowly and
release slowly. Keep your head as close to the floor as possible.*

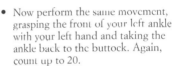

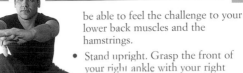

be able to feel the challenge to your lower back muscles and the hamstrings.

- Stand upright. Grasp the front of your right ankle with your right hand. Take your bent leg back until you can touch your right buttock with the sole of your right foot. Hold for 20.

For a trim bottom, work the buttock muscles and inner thigh muscles as shown above.

- Now perform the same movement, grasping the front of your left ankle with your left hand and taking the ankle back to the buttock. Again, count up to 20.
- Now do the leg stretches shown as part of the cool-down exercises described on pp 72–75, then follow these with the other cool-down exercises.

Strong, shapely calves and thighs need constant stretching and toning. Grasp first one foot with both hands and pull as close to your body as possible, and then the other. Repeat several times. Keep your back as straight as possible.

Sit ups

Sit-ups, or abdominal crunches, are best done as part of a balanced exercise programme to enhance your fitness for other activities, such as riding and squash, but can also be regarded as an exercise activity in their own right.

Some experts believe that muscle weakness in the abdomen is one of the main reasons for back pain and injury. The abdominal muscles should act as a support for the lower back. However, if those muscles are weak, too much strain may be exerted on the muscles of the lower back. Doing sit ups strengthens these muscles.

When performing sit-ups it is important not to place undue stress on either your back or your neck. The pictures below show variations on the basic sit-up described above and involve varying levels of difficulty.

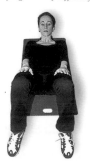
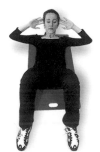

FACTFILE

Calories burnt per minute: 4.8

Benefits: abdominal strength and endurance

Works on: heart, lungs, arms, shoulders and legs

Lie with both feet placed on the floor, hands behind your head or by your sides. Your knees should be bent to avoid stress to your back. Tuck your chin down into your chest and at the same time slowly raise your upper body to meet your knees. Now slowly resume your lying position. Avoid arching your back as you lie down.

Women should aim to build up to sets of between 15 and 35 while men should be able to build up to 30–75.

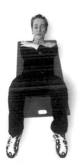
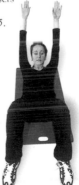

Aquaerobics

Aerobic exercise performed in water, known as aquaerobics, constitutes perfect exercise for the unfit. This is because the water supports your weight, making the risk of injury minimal. Standing in the pool, you push against the water to build up strength.

You don't need to be able to swim to practise aquaerobics – simply stay in the shallow end of the pool and let the swimmers take the middle and the deep end.

The range and type of exercises you do at an aquaerobics class (most swimming pools run them) will depend on your instructor. They are likely to include some of the following:

- the warm-up exercises described on pp 68–71
- running on the spot
- cycling or jumping on the spot
- stretching exercises
- kicking exercises, sometimes with you holding a floating board

STRETCHING EXERCISES

These are particularly effective when carried out in water because they allow you to go through a routine of exercises that stretch your muscles, so increasing your flexibility and suppleness while avoiding any undue stress and strain thanks to the support that the water provides.

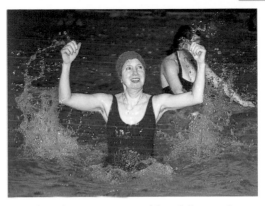

It's safe, it's fun, it's invigorating and, best of all, aquaerobics challenges all the muscles of the body while the water supports your weight. Ideal for children, the elderly and pregnant women.

Put your left hand on the edge of the pool while standing side on. Keep your back straight and raise your right leg in front of you so it is fully extended, with your big toe pointing straight ahead. Now take your right leg slowly round to your right side, pause and continue taking your leg as far back to the right as you can.

Do this 5 times.

Now repeat the sequence with your right hand on the edge of the pool and your left leg fully extended.

Do this 5 times.

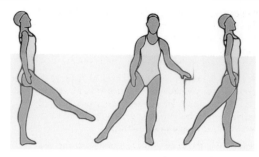

The exercises you perform in aquaerobics are much the same as you would do in an exercise class: the difference is that you can increase flexibility and suppleness much more in water than you can out of water, because the water is taking your weight.

Repeat the sequences. After a few times you should be able to feel a good stretch in the buttock muscles and the muscles of the thighs and calves. This exercise will also have a beneficial effect on your abdominal and back muscles.

Now put your left hand on the edge of the pool and sweep your right arm through a full arc. Repeat this several times.

Then, with your right hand supporting you on the edge of the pool, swing your left arm through a wide arc in the same way.

Do this several times.

You can now combine the two exercises described above so that with your left hand on the edge of the pool, you now extend your right arm and your right leg fully. Then turn round, place your right hand on the edge and fully extend your left arm and leg.

Holding on to the edge of the pool, make for the deeper water so that you are out of your depth. Maintaining your hold on the edge, let your hands take the full weight of your body, allowing the muscles to stretch downward throughout your body.

Maintaining the same position as above, bring your feet up as close to your hands as possible and stretch out your back muscles. Make sure that your upper arms are fully stretched out as well so that they too benefit.

Aquaerobic exercises can be done on your own or with a friend at your local swimming pool, or in an aquaerobics class supervised by a trained instructor. Once you have finished your exercises, and providing you are not too tired, you can have a relaxing swim.

FACTFILE

Calories burnt per minute: 5

Works on: flexibility and strength in the arms, legs, abdominal muscles, buttocks and back

Complementary exercises: cycling, walking, jogging, running, weights

Swimming

Regular swimming is an excellent method of achieving and maintaining all-round fitness. It uses all the muscle groups of the body and enhances muscular, cardiovascular and respiratory fitness. It is an especially good form of exercise because the body weight is totally supported by the water, which reduces the risk of strain or damage to your joints or muscles. For this reason, it is an activity that can be enjoyed by elderly people and those with back or other physical problems.

If you cannot swim, don't turn over the page just yet. You can learn to swim at any age and most local baths offer swimming lessons. Make it easy for yourself by getting a timetable from your local pool and keeping it on the fridge door. Some pools offer season tickets, which are cheaper than individual tickets.

You need to swim continuously and vigorously for about 10 minutes to get any benefit at all and, ideally, you need to swim at a reasonable pace for up to 30 minutes on three days of the week to achieve a good level of fitness. However, two sessions a week will still produce a noticeable benefit. Your body will become toned, with better posture and more flexibility. After only a couple of weeks you should notice the difference in your stomach muscles and shoulder muscles.

It is best to vary your stroke between breaststroke, crawl, backstroke, and butterfly. If you know only one or two strokes, why not invest in a few lessons to make

FACTFILE

Calories burnt per minute (based on swimming 18 m/20yds a minute): front crawl 4.5–5.4; backstroke 3.5–4.3; breaststroke 4.5–5.4

Benefits: strength, endurance, flexibility, mobility

Works on: arms, stomach, shoulders, back and legs

Complementary exercises: weight/circuit training

You need: pool entrance fees, swimming costume, towel, goggles and kickboard (optional)

your trips more interesting as well as more rewarding in fitness terms.

You can monitor your progress and achievements when you swim at a pool by keeping a note of how many lengths you do every 20 minutes or every 30 minutes.

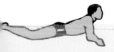 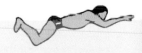

One of the advantages of swimming is that the water bears your weight and this makes it particularly attractive for overweight people and for pregnant women. Breaststroke, shown here, generally uses more muscle groups of all the strokes.

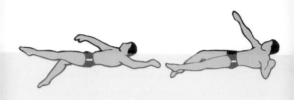

*In backstroke, shown above, it is important that your head is
well back in the water and that you make the maximum effort
with your arms and legs in order to increase your fitness in
muscular, cardiovascular and respiratory terms.*

EXERCISES TO DO IN THE POOL

- Tread water out of your depth for about 10 minutes,
  pushing your legs down and out.

- Take a deep breath and push yourself down to the
  bottom of the pool, then push yourself up while you
  are breathing out (respiratory benefit).

- Swim one length as fast as you can, then swim slowly
  back (or get out of the pool and walk back to the
  start). Repeat several times.

- Hold the edge of the pool with outstretched arms,
  assume the front crawl position with your head
  immersed in the water. Kick with your legs as you
  count to five, turn your head to the side and breathe
  in, return your head to the water and keep kicking.

Never swim directly after eating. Allow at least 2 hours
to elapse after a heavy meal.

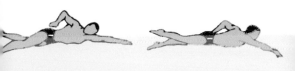

Freestyle or crawl is a fast and rhythmic stroke that exercises all the main muscles of the body. It can be a racing style or a slow endurance stroke. Technique is all-important, and it may be worth investing in a few lessons at your local swimming pool to perfect not only your stroke but also your breathing technique. It is important to keep your head down, with the water surface at the line between your forehead and hair. Breathe in and out as your head is turned to the side.

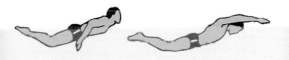

The butterfly stroke demands more physical effort than the other swimming strokes, but it more than repays the investment in terms of the benefit it brings to your cardiorespiratory fitness, as well as to upper body strength and increased flexibility. Some lessons will prove valuable if you have not yet mastered this powerful stroke.

Step exercise

Step exercise is a concentrated and effective means of developing your leg muscles and of increasing your respiratory and cardiovascular fitness (it can therefore be described as an aerobic exercise).

Step exercise also promotes agility as the speed at which you are able to change your body position and direction increases. Speed and agility, in turn, depend on your strength and endurance. The repetitive nature of step exercise means that you can devote your entire energy to it and the more

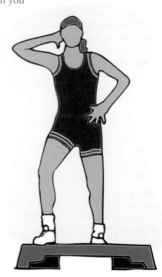

Your step may be made of rigid foam, plastic or wood. Improvise if necessary, but make sure that your step is safe before you start exercising.

you put into it, of course – as with any type of exercise – the more you will get out of it.

You simply step up, down, up, down, right, left, right, left, right, right, left, left, left, down, up, down in a number of different sequences and patterns. You can increase your speed and/or the length of time you devote to step exercise in accordance with your increasing level of fitness and muscular control.

Most gyms, health clubs and centres run step classes, which are good to attend because they help to motivate you, maintain a good pace and make performing the exercise more fun. Classes usually last between 30 and 50 minutes. Plastic steps are generally used, although steps can also be made of blocks of wood or firm foam. Steps vary in height: the higher the step, the greater the cardiovascular and respiratory benefit.

You can also do step exercises at home. Use the bottom step of the stairs, the front or back doorstep or a firm box. Step exercises are often done to music as this helps to get a rhythm going. You can then add arm movements (see illustration opposite) to increase your cardiovascular effort and further develop your fitness.

After your warm-up exercises (see pp 68–71), start with sessions of 10 minutes a day several times a week, gradually increasing up to 25 minutes a day on five days of the week. This is all you need to do to achieve and maintain fitness. It is so simple. When you finish your session, always remember to do some stretch and cool-down exercises (see pp 72–75).

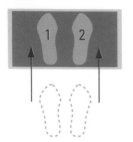 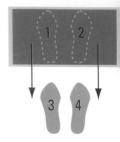

YOU CAN VARY YOUR STEP PATTERNS IN A NUMBER OF WAYS

1 Basic step: step up with your left foot. Step down. Step up with your right foot. Step down. Repeat. Step up with your right foot. Step down. Step up with your left foot. Step down. Repeat.

2 Step up with your left foot. Bring your right foot up to the step, keeping a hips' width between your feet. Step with your right foot to the right. Draw the left foot up to the right. Step to the left with your left foot. Draw your right foot up to the left. Step down. Repeat.

Now repeat this in the opposite direction as follows:

3 Step up with your right foot. Bring your left foot up to the step, keeping your feet apart. Step with your

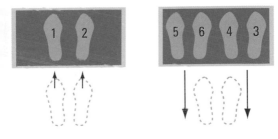

left foot to the left. Draw the right foot up to the left. Step to the right with your right foot. Draw your left foot up to the right. Step down. Repeat.

As you become more skilled and more in time with the music, you will be able to increase your pace. Aim to do 40 step ups with each foot without stopping.

FACTFILE

Calories burnt per minute: 13

Works on: strength, stamina and endurance in the legs; increases speed and agility

Complementary exercises: weight training, swimming, walking

Skipping

This is a wonderful exercise that uses all the main muscle groups of the body and also enhances your cardiovascular and respiratory fitness. It strengthens and tones the muscles, is an excellent way of warming up before other exercises and is also useful training for sports requiring stamina, coordination and rhythm, such as boxing, athletics and weight training.

Start with 10 minutes of warm-up exercises before you skip. Always skip on a level piece of ground so that any strain on the body is evenly distributed through your legs and thighs in order to avoid injury.

HOW TO SKIP

- Keep your back straight and your head facing forward.
- Breathe through your nose.
- Keep the rope turning as smoothly as possible using your wrists and forearms.

When you start skipping you may be surprised at how testing it is given that it looks so easy and relaxing. You may become quickly out of breath, but don't be discouraged, your respiratory fitness levels will soon rise to cope with the extra workload – to your benefit.

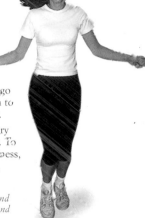

- Push off with your toes.
- Bend your knees and jump only so high as to clear the rope, no higher.
- Land lightly on the balls of your feet.
- After five minutes, make the rope go in the opposite direction to ensure all-round benefit.

Skipping 5–15 minutes every day will get you into shape. To maintain a good level of fitness, aim to skip for 20 minutes, three times a week.

As you skip, relax your neck and shoulders. Maintain an even and regular breathing rate.

FACTFILE

Calories burnt per minute: 4.8

Works on: strengthening chest and buttocks; neck, arm/leg muscles, shoulders, good for posture

Complementary exercises: swimming, walking

Badminton

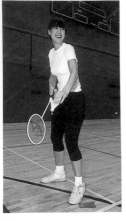

Weather poses no problem with badminton. Your local library or local council will be able to give you information about your nearest courts or club.

Your strength and stamina are bound to improve if you play badminton on a regular basis. However, like tennis, it is not the best of aerobic sports because you are not moving continuously for any length of time. To achieve a good level of fitness, try combining badminton with brisk walking, running or vigorous swimming.

Badminton demands perfect body control with everything synchronized for the ideal stroke: good balance, knees bent, body leaning into the stroke, elbow bent, correct grip, early and full back-swing and, vitally, eyes on the shuttlecock from the second it leaves your opponent's racquet. Your footwork demands good braking, quick starting, bending, stretching, turning, jumping and instantaneous changes of direction. Once you join a club, you will be able to improve your serve, learn

FACTFILE

Calories burnt per minute: 5.1–6.2 (singles); 3.8–4.6 (social doubles)

Works on: strength and flexibility in the arms, legs, shoulders, back and abdomen; good for coordination

You need: light and flexible shoes with some interior cushioning. They should have a soft but rough or ridged light-coloured sole to give you grip for stopping and turning. Lacing should go from toe to instep and the tongue should be lightly padded. A padded heel tab support can prevent problems with your Achilles tendon.

variations on the serve technique, how to perfect your forehand, backhand, drop shot, smash and other techniques, as well as gaining an insight into forcing your opponent into making errors.

Don't forget to do your warm-up and cool-down exercises (see pp 68–75).

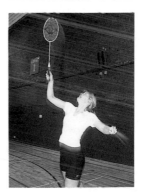

Stretching for overhead shots helps improve flexibility.

Tennis

Tennis is an excellent way of achieving and maintaining a certain level of fitness. It is not of such aerobic value as other sports because it is not a sustained activity. However, playing tennis improves your muscular strength and endurance and develops balance and hand-to-eye coordination. Singles is a far more strenuous game than doubles.

It is important that you first do some warm-up exercises (see pp 68–71) and some stretch 'n' tone exercises (see pp 82–85) before starting a game of tennis in order to avoid straining the muscles.

Good technique in tennis is important for improving your game and to avoid injury. It is best to learn tennis as a child, although you can pay for lessons through tennis clubs and some health and fitness centres. Classes are available for beginners, refreshers and children.

You can then practise alone or with a partner, working on your serve and volley and on your forehand and backhand actions.

Tennis is an attractive and sociable way of keeping fit, particularly in the summer months. Municipal courts can be booked and racquet hire is available. Many clubs now keep their courts open in the daylight hours of the winter and use floodlights as it gets darker. You will also find that some clubs have indoor courts, so you needn't lose your match fitness during the winter months.

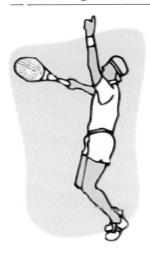

The tennis serve challenges your muscular strength and flexibility. You need good leg muscles and strong shoulders and forearms to deliver a powerful serve. Working with weights helps to develop the shoulders and makes a good complement to tennis.

FACTFILE

Calories burnt per minute. 7–8.5 (singles); 4.8–5.9 (doubles)

Works on: mobility, strength, endurance and flexibility in the arms, shoulders, back, abdomen and legs

Complementary exercises: weights, swimming

Riding

Riding is aerobic exercise and develops muscular, cardiovascular and respiratory fitness. There are different types of horse riding, some of which make greater demands on your body than others.

When your mount is walking, your leg muscles, particularly your calves, are constantly active as you make contact with its girth and nudge it along with the back of your ankles. As you go into a trot, your leg muscles continue to grip the horse's girth but now your body is faced with the additional challenge of rising from the knees in your seat – up, down, up, down, repeatedly, using your calves and knees as you push off from the saddle. Once you are into a canter, you no longer rise in the saddle, but your leg grip needs to be powerful if you are to stay astride.

FACTFILE

Calories burnt per minute: 2.9–8.7

Benefits: good for muscular endurance in the legs and stimulates cardiorespiratory fitness

Complementary exercises: swimming, aerobics

You need: safety helmet, riding boots, riding gloves (rubber-coated string gloves), especially in the rain as wet reins are difficult to grip

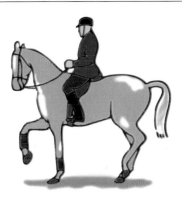

Riding is particularly good for developing your coordination and balance, and because of this it is of benefit to your posture. It is also good for the muscular fitness of your legs and upper body. Ideally, you should learn to ride when you are still a child as children find it easier than adults to adjust to the rhythm of the horse and develop a natural seat.

PRE-RIDING EXERCISES FOR EXTRA SUPPLENESS AND POWER

- Lean forward over the horse's neck to touch your left toe with your right hand. Now repeat the process on the other side. Continue until you feel limbered up.

- With arms outstretched, and head up and slightly back, turn around as far as possible, twisting your upper body from the hips. This is designed to increase the suppleness of your back and waist.

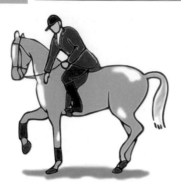

Warm up for 10 minutes before you mount so that you are using your legs and hands to full effect from the minute you are astride rather than 5 or 10 minutes later.

- In order to loosen up your back muscles, fold your arms over your chest and lean right back on to the horse's quarters, with your legs remaining in the normal riding position.

Buying and owning a horse can be very expensive but you can hire them quite easily. Once you have learned to ride, the options are unlimited:

- hacking out once or twice a week with a riding school (trotting, cantering, galloping and jumping in a variety of terrains)
- showjumping (taking the horse over a series of different types of jumps in competition)
- dressage (taking the horse through a series of specific and carefully controlled manoeuvres)

- cross-country trials (timed competitions over set courses with a number of different styles of jump)
- riding holidays in which you trek several miles a day (a good introduction to horse riding for beginners)
- mountain-trail riding (a group trek along a trail in mountainous countryside)

It is best to learn to ride with a qualified instructor at a British Horse Society-approved riding school (see Useful addresses). The cost of riding will vary from area to area. As a rough guide, individual lessons can range from £8–£20, whereas hacking in a group, for example, will be less costly. You should always, without exception, wear a safety hat.

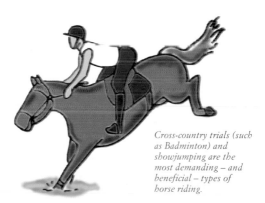

Cross-country trials (such as Badminton) and showjumping are the most demanding – and beneficial – types of horse riding.

Cycling

Riding a bicycle requires more muscular effort and cardiovascular endurance than walking, and is especially good for the legs. Mountain biking off-road has the added advantage of working the upper body muscles. If cycling is your chosen exercise, complement it with some upper body work such as working with weights, squash, swimming the crawl or golf.

With more towns now having cycle lanes it's easier to ride instead of taking the car or using public transport. The more you cycle, the further you will be able to ride. This is best done on a regular and sustained basis, making your bicycle a part of everyday life. For real benefit, aim to cycle 15–20 minutes a day at 16kph/10mph. You should be able to cycle 8kph/5 miles in approximately 30–35 minutes or 16kph/10 miles in 1 hour.

FACTFILE

Calories burnt per minute: 8.1–9.8 (based on cycling at 16kph/10mph)

Works on: improving the endurance of the upper and lower legs; excellent cardiovascular exercise

Complementary exercises: walking, jogging, weights, squash, front crawl, golf, weight training

You need: bike, safety helmet, fluorescent strip

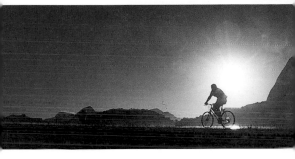

Cycling into the sunset after an afternoon's brisk ride must surely be one of the great pleasures of life. Cycling cannot be improved upon for its benefit to the heart muscles and the muscles of the thighs and calves.

Other types of cycling include track and road racing, both only for the very fit. Track racing is a competitive sport and requires a special bike and banked track. In road-racing, long distances (up to hundreds of kilometres) are covered on a lightweight bike. Mountain biking can be enjoyed by everyone; the sturdy frame of mountain bikes allow you to take them over the toughest terrain (although this requires some hard cycling). Or why not join a cycling club where you will find people of all ages cycling for fun?

Of course, if you want to cycle without leaving home, there are stationary cycling machines. The intensity of exercise on these machines can be easily controlled.

Working with weights

Weight or resistance training is probably the ideal way
of developing muscular fitness (improvements in
respiratory and cardiovascular fitness are seen but are
not as great). Despite its often bad press, weight
training is safe, effective and can be very enjoyable.
Although it is possible to train at home, it is more
sensible (and fun) to attend a gym. Here you can be
assessed for your fitness level and expectations, and also

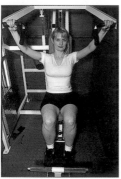

*Grasping the handles, pull
down on the bar until it
touches the back of your
neck. Then slowly let the bar
rise to its full extension.*

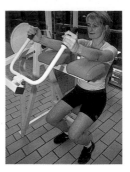

*With your elbows on each
pad, push the bar away from
you using the muscles in your
arms. The use of machines
instead of free weights
reduces the risk of injury.*

be shown how to use the equipment safely and effectively. Most gyms have a combination of free-weights (barbells and dumbbells) and resistance machines. An instructor will also be on hand to give advice and devise a training programme to suit your needs.

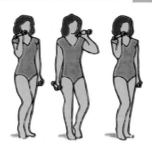

You can walk or run with hand-held weights. Raise the weight in one hand to shoulder level, keeping the other by your side and alternate as you walk.

Always warm up thoroughly prior to weight training and do some cool-down exercises once you have finished.

When performing weight training exercises it is important to use a smooth, steady continuous motion. Avoid jerking the movements. If lifting weights, always raise the weights slowly and then slowly return them to their resting position.

A typical example of a basic training routine would include one exercise for each body part (chest, back, shoulders, arms and legs). Each exercise would then be performed for three sets of 10–12 repetitions. Ideally, routines should be performed three times a week for 30 minutes to an hour. Once your confidence and ability improve you can increase either the weight you are

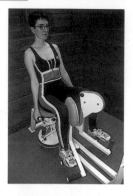

Sitting comfortably on the chair and grasping the handles, place your knees on the outside of each paddle. Using a smooth motion, bring your knees together using the muscles of your inner thighs.

lifting or the number of repetitions you are doing.

It is very important when you first start weight training not to overdo it. Your body and muscles will not be used to such focused attention and it is very easy to 'over-train' or strain yourself. You will not become a bodybuilder overnight – it takes years of hard training to develop muscles and lift bigger weights. Take it easy and have fun.

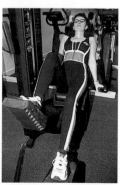

Sitting with your back firmly against the board and hands holding the grips, place your feet against the paddles and push down with alternate feet using your thigh muscles.

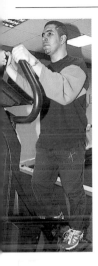

Before working out with weights, even small hand-held ones (below), it is important that you warm up your muscles thoroughly A step machine is ideal for this. Use it by grasping the handles firmly, and pushing down on the foot plates in a stepping motion.

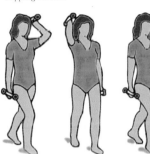

FACTFILE

Calories burnt per minute: 7.3

Works on: muscular endurance and strength in the arms, chest, back, shoulders and legs

Complementary exercises: aerobics, circuit training, step exercise, boxing, rowing, swimming, walking

You need: a variety of weights, proper supervision

Jogging and running

Both are excellent forms of aerobic exercise and very good for improving stamina and general muscular strength in the lower part of the body, as well as greatly improving your lung efficiency.

To be effective aerobic exercise, you need to get up into your training zone (see pp 60–61). You should aim to jog or run for anything up to an hour several times a week. You could run for 30 minutes on five days of the week or 50 minutes on three days of the week. Most experts advise us not to run or jog every day so that the body has a chance to rest and the opportunity to repair itself. Eventually, once you have built up enough stamina and strength, you may like to start taking part in longer runs such as 10km runs, half or even full marathons.

Warm-up exercises are a must before jogging or running as are cool-down exercises when you finish. Always drink a glass of water or two before you start and again when

FACTFILE

Calories burnt per minute: 8.5–10.3 (based on running at 8kph/5mph)

Works on: cardiorespiratory fitness and benefits the arms, legs, chest and abdominal muscles

Complementary exercises: swimming, weights

you finish in order to replace lost body fluids. Eat a well-balanced diet (see pp 34–41), especially carbohydrates.

RUNNING TIPS

• Breathe rhythmically through your mouth and inhale deeply from your abdomen.

• Keep your head up, back straight and buttocks tucked under, arms swinging to balance your movements.

• Set an even pace, with a short stride, from the hips.

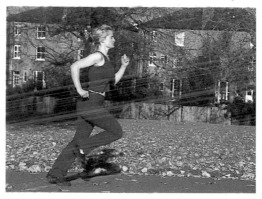

Your arms are an important aid to fitness as you run or jog. Focus on your shoulders so that they are relaxed. Allow your arms to swing, so that when one is stretched backward the other is stretched well forward. Avoid dipping your head and stretching your neck out in front of you – look straight ahead.

Circuit training

Circuit training is used to develop all-round strength, fitness and muscular endurance. It is used by athletes to complement their existing training regimes although, even by itself, it is a very effective means of getting fit.

Circuits are designed to suit an individual's needs and will vary depending on what each person is trying to accomplish. They are often used by athletes to improve their performance in a particular field. For example, a 100-metre sprinter would tailor a circuit to increase explosive power. The focus here is on lower body development. A rower, on the other hand, would concentrate on developing upper body strength, cardiovascular and respiratory fitness.

A basic circuit combines several different exercises performed in rotation. Once all the exercises have been performed, the circuit is complete. Exercises can be

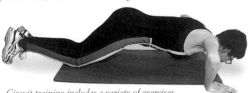

Circuit training includes a variety of exercises designed to strengthen the upper body, the shoulders, the arms and the legs. When you work against resistance, as shown here, your cardiovascular and muscular effort increase, which benefits your fitness levels.

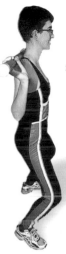

Incorporating work with weights into your circuit training will increase your muscular strength and stamina.

performed in combinations of sets and repetitions (a set is a certain number of repetitions of a particular exercise). As fitness increases you can adapt the circuit; adding to it, increasing the number of sets and circuits performed and decreasing the time taken to perform each circuit.

Circuit training is a popular method of general fitness and includes exercises for the chest, shoulders, back, arms and legs. It is excellent for muscular fitness and builds up cardiovascular and respiratory endurance. Many sports centres have weekly group classes, where an instructor will set out a basic circuit that the participants follow. Each session lasts approximately 30 minutes. Circuits can be changed on a regular basis to prevent boredom and keep you challenged.

FACTFILE

Calories burnt per minute: 13.6

Works on: shoulders, stomach, back, arms and legs

Aerobic exercise

To many people, the word 'aerobics' means an energetic exercise class in a gym. But in fact, aerobic (which literally means 'with oxygen') exercises are any sustained activities that result in an increase of oxygenated blood to all the muscles and organs of the body. This means that all those sports that require continuous activity and boost the heart rate and breathing, for example, jogging, running, swimming, rowing, cycling and brisk walking, are very beneficial and effective aerobic activities.

When any aerobic exercise is performed on a regular basis, it can improve stamina and endurance. To reap maximum benefit from aerobic exercise, you have to be working within your training zone, that is, any continuous activity that pushes your heart rate up to between 60 and 90% of the maximum rate for your age (see pp 60–61).

Aerobic exercise need not be a hard slog – in fact it is not advisable to push

Once you have learned a good variety of aerobic exercises in a class that is suitable for your age and level of fitness, you will be able to continue at home for 20 minutes a day on five days of the week, thus ensuring an excellent level of fitness.

yourself too hard – although you do need to make some physical effort to derive any benefit. Aim to build up the level of activity gradually. Once you start to become aerobically fit, you will find your exercise sessions less tiring and your normal day far less exhausting in general.

You should aim for between 20 and 60 minutes on three to five days of the week for optimum fitness. This should be done at between 60 and 90% of your normal maximum heart rate.

Anaerobic exercise, incidentally, means exercise without oxygen: you are calling on short bursts of energy as you would in, for example, sprinting or squash. Anaerobic exercise helps to develop muscular strength, but it should be used only as a supplement to aerobic exercise once you are fit.

Running is an excellent aerobic activity, whether you are exercising on a treadmill, jogging in the park, or running longer distances.

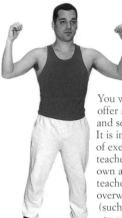

Running with your arms above your head increases your respiratory effort and enhances your fitness tremendously.

AEROBICS CLASSES

You will find aerobics classes on offer at leisure centres, health centres and some adult education institutes. It is important to learn a good variety of exercises from an experienced teacher before continuing with your own aerobic sessions at home. The teacher will ensure that you do not overwork certain parts of the body (such as knee joints) and will be able to adjust the speed and intensity of the class to the appropriate level of fitness.

There are two types of aerobics classes: low-impact and high-impact. Both involve similar kinds of exercises, but high-impact aerobics classes provide better cardiovascular exercise. Classes in general last between 30 and 50 minutes and will consist of many different exercises, all of which are designed to work on various parts of the body. A typical aerobics class might include: jogging/running on the spot, jumping up and down, upper body work using dumbbells and bars, waist twists, lower body work, including squatting, leg and

Your starting pose for side stretches, twists and bends – all of which are excellent for limbering up and for developing the oblique abdominal muscles.

calf raises, star jumps, lunges, kicks, sit ups and bottom crunches. The aim is to keep on the move for most of the time.

Music is an integral part of any aerobics session; it helps to motivate the class, keep up or vary the pace and makes the class more lively and enjoyable. You can, of course, buy your own tapes, CDs or videotapes for use at home.

FACTFILE

Calories burnt per minute: 8.5

Works on: arms (biceps/triceps), legs, stomach muscles, waist, chest and buttocks

Complementary exercises: weight/circuit training, swimming, walking, yoga

Gymnastics

Gymnastics can involve work with the vault, the beam, the wall bars, and with apparatus such as the rope, the hoop, the ribbon and stick, the ball and a set of clubs. However, body work is the basis of good gymnastics. Floor exercises such as turning, leaping, lunging and rolling all require a high level of fitness, so if it is optimum fitness that you desire, then gymnastics makes an excellent choice. It is a good exercise for children and anyone who is still naturally supple but is not generally suitable for the over-60s.

Before you start your gymnastic practice, it is always important that you go through a series of warm-up exercises (see pp 68–71) for 5–10 minutes in order to stretch your muscles and increase your suppleness. This is vital because it will help to reduce the danger of injury.

The fundamental techniques you will learn at a class at your local gym are:

1 Swinging and circling

2 Throwing and catching

In swinging you need to transfer your body weight from one foot to the other in a smooth movement, while at the same time managing the piece of equipment that you are using. In circling, a circular movement is performed with various apparatus, such as ribbon.

Throwing and catching balls, hoops and clubs requires

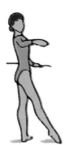
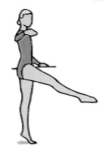

The basic positions learned in women's gymnastics are very similar to ballet postures, both demanding the development of skill, agility and grace.

you to be sufficiently coordinated to perform a single, double or even triple forward roll while at the same time managing, for example, the hoop or the clubs.

You will learn how to spin, roll, rotate, toss, juggle and bounce the various pieces of equipment using your feet, legs, shoulders and back to balance your weight.

Footwork is, of course, of the utmost importance in gymnastics. Your footwork needs to be intricate, precise and well-defined. Indeed, you will see that many of the steps used are derived from classical ballet (see illustrations above). As you progress both in technique and in fitness you will move on to different types of leaps, jumps and turns.

Muscular fitness is challenged to the full in the balance

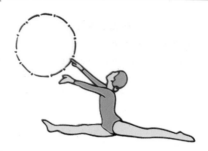

Advanced gymnastics involves postures such as the splits combined with the use of equipment (known as apparatus), including the hoop.

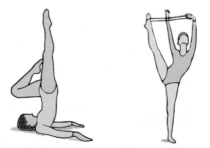

Optimum muscular fitness and balance in the shoulders, forearms and abdomen are required to hold this striking pose (left) and this one with the additional use of apparatus (right).

FACTFILE

Calories burnt per minute: 3.3–5

Benefits: strength, endurance, suppleness and flexibility

Works on: arms, legs, buttocks, stomach, chest, shoulders, back and neck

positions (see illustrations opposite). Body waves (a fluid movement along the body that gives the appearance of a 'ripple') can be a spectacular sight. Back bends (stretching slowly backward until the hands and arms are resting on the floor and the back is arched) should be carried out with care and only when you are fully fit. Sit ups are an excellent method of preparation for the back bend because they strengthen the abdominal muscles that support the back and protect it from injury.

Acrobatics form part of the spectacle of gymnastics when performed at the highest level. Some types of gymnastics include the handstand, the cartwheel, the handspring and the somersault.

The integration of tempo and rhythm is now an essential part of gymnastics, bringing the sport ever closer to modern dance.

Training for gymnastics requires many hours to be spent in developing strength, flexibility and stamina. Some experts believe that the single most important component in successful gymnastics is strength.

Squash

Squash is an extremely high-energy sport, much more so than tennis, and uses up some 600 calories an hour. You need to be fit and supple for squash. It is all too easy for untrained muscles to be badly strained and damaged due to the speed of the game and the twisting movements involved. Therefore, to make the most of squash, you need to have achieved a good level of fitness before you start playing. For example, walking and running, or cycling, are perfect complementary exercises to the type of muscular actions and levels of fitness required for squash. These rhythmic activities are sustained and thus enhance your cardiovascular and respiratory fitness.

Ideally, have some coaching from a squash professional because it is important to move around the court properly. (You should be able to arrange lessons at your local squash club quite easily.) With an improved technique, the risk of injury is lower, your game will improve and so will your enjoyment and fitness.

In order to sustain peak level fitness, you need to play three times a week all year round. Always start with a glass of water, a good 10 minutes' of warm-up exercises (pp 68–71) and then some stretch 'n' tone exercises (pp 82–85) to maximize your suppleness. When you finish playing, put on a fleece or sweater and drink some more water: because squash is so strenuous, your body will cool down quickly when you finish.

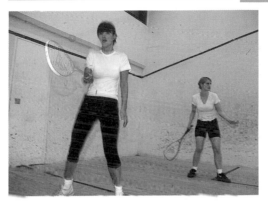

The keynote here is to be fit before you start in order to avoid the all-too common injuries caused by the speed of the game. Walking, running and working with weights will all prove useful. Invest in some lessons in order to develop your game and minimize the risk of injury.

FACTFILE

Calories burnt per minute: 9.5–11.5

Works on: legs, arms, shoulders, back and abdomen; increases speed, mobility, strength, endurance and flexibility

You need: proper squash shoes, squash racquet, ball

Rowing

Rowing is a pleasurable and energetic, even strenuous activity that you can do either as an individual or as part of a team with perhaps Olympic ambitions.

If you join a rowing club, you must be able to provide evidence that you can swim – you can obtain a certificate through your local swimming pool.

You will learn how to handle the boat, how to place it in the water, how to get into the boat, the correct way to hold an oar, how to row and how to get out of the boat.

Rowing is a vigorous sport that provides excellent, all-round exercise and promotes strength and stamina. It is especially good for developing the upper body, without overdeveloping the shoulders. Rowing is not harmful to the back unless there is some pre-existing injury or weakness.

Because rowing is a strenuous activity, training and diet are all important. Training continues through the winter, in the rain and cold and on rough water created by strong wind conditions. Sessions vary and may last from one hour a week to two hours a day depending on your level of ability and interest. It focuses on:

- Increasing muscle efficiency
- Improving mental skills (encouraging self-belief)
- Increasing technical ability (to reduce the muscular effort made)

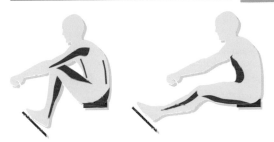

The rowing stroke comprises four phases: the catch (shown left), as the oar dips into the water; the leg drive (shown right); the finish, as you push the water away from you in order to propel the boat; and the recovery to starting position, where the arms straighten, the trunk rotates forward and the legs bend.

Training can also be done on rowing machines that have stationary or sliding seats. The principle is the same – the legs are exercised in a bending and pulling movement and the chest and arms are strengthened.

As you can see from the illustrations above, the rowing stroke requires tremendous muscular effort.

FACTFILE

Calories burnt per minute: 5

Works on: arms, shoulders, chest, stomach, legs

Complementary exercises: walking, swimming

Boxing

Boxing demands a combination of strength, stamina, coordination, agility and speed – you have to be 100 per cent fit, whatever your level.

Your upper body has to be strong enough to absorb punches, while at the same time you must have the muscular endurance to be able to punch effectively. Your shoulders and upper arms have to be strong and powerful and you

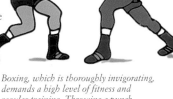

Boxing, which is thoroughly invigorating, demands a high level of fitness and regular training. Throwing a punch demands considerable coordination and suppleness, strength in the upper body and speed on the legs.

also need to be fast and agile with the endurance to get through several rounds.

Boxers do a lot of skipping exercises (see pp 100–101) as part of their training regime. This increases their muscular strength and endurance, cardiorespiratory endurance, flexibility, agility, balance and footwork. Shadow boxing (sparring without a partner) is used to improve reflexes, technique and coordination.

The five-stage syllabus issued by the Amateur Boxing Association of England Ltd includes:

1 Stance/guard/footwork

- Correct positioning of the feet
- Compact guard with hands held in a position to attack, defend or counter
- Ability to move forward or backward without upsetting balance

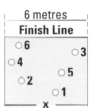

You will learn to move quickly and accurately, dancing around your partner, as shown in the numbered steps above, while at the same time throwing a powerful punch.

2 Jab to head and body with defences against

3 Use of the rear hand and defences

4 Combination punching

5 Flair and self-expression

A contentious sport from a medical point of view, boxing must always be professionally supervised.

FACTFILE

Benefits: cardiovascular and muscular endurance, strength and flexibility in all areas

Complementary exercises: running, aerobics, weight/circuit training, step exercise

Movement and dance

Any type of rhythmic movement and dance will benefit you in terms of muscular, respiratory and cardiovascular fitness. It is also good for increasing stamina levels, posture and movement control. Dance classes, while providing fantastic exercise for the heart, lungs and muscles, are also fun and a great way to unwind. For many, music is one of the great pleasures of life, and thus fitness through this sort of exercise becomes even more of a positive pleasure.

You will find many different dance classes on offer at your local adult education centre and some may also be available privately in your area. Check out the options.

- Jazz dance
- Dancexercise (a cross between an aerobics class and dance)
- Modern dance (contemporary ballet)
- Tap dance
- Ballet
- Ballroom dancing
- Line dancing (see pp 136–139)
- Belly dancing (see pp 140–143)
- Flamenco (Spanish dancing)
- Scottish country dancing

- Greek dancing
- Latin American dance (e.g. salsa – see pp 144–147 – cha cha, samba, rumba, tango)
- Morris dance
- Jive

Never be afraid to join a beginners' class. Dance classes are usually great fun, and are a good way of socializing and achieving fitness. And the more you practise at home, on your own or with a friend, the better for your fitness and style.

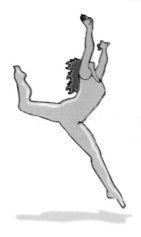

Modern dance requires strength and grace: find a local beginner's class in order to develop technique and style.

FACTFILE

Calories burnt per minute: 6.3

Works on: arms, legs, buttocks and stomach; increases strength, stamina and suppleness; good for posture and movement

Line dancing

If you like country-and-western music and you like dancing, then this is the very best way of achieving and maintaining fitness.

Line dancing has become a fantastically popular national craze in the United Kingdom in the 1990s. Village halls all over the country are putting on weekly class/club sessions – and it has proved to be almost as popular with men as it is with women.

Line dancing is essentially country-and-western dancing in drill lines, and sometimes in a circle. Line dancing has its own etiquette, its own distinctive footwork (it is made up of a number of different steps each with its own name) and characteristic body stances. It does not matter how fit you are when you start line dancing – you can do two or three dances and then sit out a dance or two to allow your breathing and muscles to recover. Although initially it might not seem as demanding as other forms of dance, it can be quite exhausting. However, as your stamina, endurance and overall fitness increase by attending weekly sessions and by practising at home to a tape or videotape, you will find that you no longer need – or want – to sit out.

Line dancing is hard to beat as regular and sustained exercise, and it is fun. What's more you do not need a partner. It is usually more fun to go line dancing with a group of single friends.

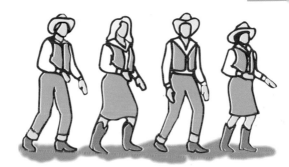

At first sight, line dancing does not look as if it would be very taxing but, in fact, it is a demanding – and rewarding – form of exercise, as well as a good night out

Part of the appeal of line dancing is the regularity and individual coordination of the lines. So you need to concentrate on which way you are meant to be facing and what steps you are doing – don't worry, you'll be told! You should stand directly behind the person in front of you, so that the front to back line is straight and you should make sure that you continue the left to right line by standing exactly next to the person on your left and the person on your right.

Footwork is the primary consideration in line dancing and at first you will probably concentrate on that to the exclusion of everything else.

As you learn the steps, however, you will start to incorporate the hip movements (rocks, bumps and swivels) and hand claps and boot slaps. The arms are of lesser importance, and women look good when both hands are clasped behind the back. Alternatively, do as the men do and hook your thumbs into your belt loops at the front of your jeans.

The following is an example of the kind of steps used:

1 Walk forward right

2&3 Walk forward left, right

4&5 Coaster step (forward left, together right, back left)

6&7 Walk backward right, left

8&9 Coaster step (backward right, together left, forward right)

10&11 Step left behind right to right side, step right to right side

The hat, the waistcoat and the cowboy boots are de rigueur. A denim skirt or figure-hugging jeans complete the picture.

12&13 Modified sailor shuffle (left behind right, right in place, left to left side)

FACTFILE

Calories burnt per minute: 6.3

Works on: legs, stomach, buttocks

You need: you can wear anything you like to go line dancing, except trainers or other rubber-soled shoes. You need shoes that have soles with some slip to them in order to perform the intricate footwork

For full effect, however, you will want to wear a cowboy hat, a check shirt, a narrow leather string tie at the collar, waistcoat, jeans or denim skirt with a leather belt and cowboy boots

14&15 Step right behind left to left side, step left to left side

16&17 Modified sailor shuffle (right behind left, left in place, right to right side)

18&19 Step left behind right to right side, step right to right side

20&21 Left shuffle forward

22&23 Walk forward right, left

24 Hitch right and clap

And you do get to holler Yee-hah!

Belly dancing

Belly dancing is a thrilling and unique way of keeping fit while at the same time injecting some glamour and fun into your life.

Belly dancing originated from a combination of symbolic rituals and sexual stimulation. The undulating movements of the pelvis and abdomen, involving considerable muscular control, are symbolic enactments of conception and birth and in many cultures constituted an essential part of religion and way of life. The health-promoting aspects of muscular fitness and respiratory fitness were incidental.

Variations of belly dancing are practised all over Africa, the Near East, Middle East and Far East, but it is in Turkey and Egypt that belly dancing is still very much a part of today's culture. In India, the belly dance movements are as much an art form as a part of religious worship. The Hawaiian hula-hula is also thought to be related to belly dancing.

Belly dancers learn how to control the stomach muscles in an inward and outward direction.

Your learning programme will include:

- Learning to breathe correctly

- Learning to move to the rhythm of the music, which is unlike Western music rhythms

- Standing exercises – side stretch, alternate side stretch, limb and body stretching, lifting and expanding the ribcage, the abdominal flutter, the abdominal lift, the abdominal roll, manipulating the ribcage, and upper body circulation

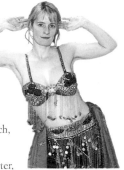

Complex but graceful arm movements help to tone up the arm muscles.

- Floor exercises – side stretch, alternate side stretch, body lift, the crescent, pelvic thrust, manipulation of the ribcage, leg strengthening, cat pose (press up), thigh and abdomen stretching

- Neck and shoulder exercises while seated

After performing these exercises, you will progress to learning the dance steps.

The dance includes:

- Basic hip rotation

- Travelling hip rotation

- Undulating hip rotation

- Hip lifts and drops
- Pelvic roll
- Figure of eight
- Pelvic tilt (in different directions)
- Camel rock, a basic step that requires you to shift the weight from one leg to the other while simultaneously contracting the abdomen and slightly arching your back

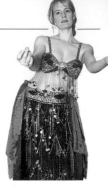

Some movements are practised while travelling, improving the coordination.

- The shimmy variations (basic, undulating, travelling, side, backbend)
- Spinning the whole body
- The characteristic head slide in which the head looks as if it is sliding on your shoulders from one side to another
  - Complex arm movements
  - Learning to dance with a veil and how to move the veil in twirling, draping and flip-over

The dancer learns to isolate different muscle groups. Here the focus is on the hips, while the top part of the body remains still.

movements as well as how to discard the veil gracefully

Once you have learned and mastered the basic techniques you will then practise putting everything together in a graceful, controlled, elegant and rhythmic style. Before long you will be able to dance with complex arm movements that are enhanced by the use of the zills, small finger cymbals, and the veil to add a touch of pizzazz to your performance. Wear a decorative bra, hip belt (in chiffon or a shiny fabric) decorated with beading, sequins, glittery braid, gold coins and chains for extra effect.

Belly dancing is becoming increasingly popular and more widely available. Look out for classes at your local adult evening institute, local library, dance schools, and Turkish and Arabic cultural centres.

Belly dancing is also good for strengthening the back muscles.

FACTFILE

Calories burnt per minute: 6.5

Works on: upper body, arms, legs, back, stomach and pelvic floor muscles; good for general posture

Salsa

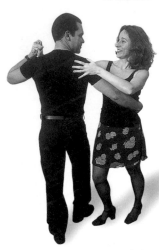

The word 'salsa' comes from *echale salsita*, meaning 'spice it up'. And that's exactly what salsa does to the diverse mixture of Latin American music styles and rhythms that have come to be known collectively as salsa. Salsa draws on guaracha danzon, cha cha cha, pachanga, rumba, mambo and others as well as new dance steps. It is an Afro-Caribbean style of dance that is constantly evolving, and for

The hot music and spicy style of salsa mean this Latin American dance demands 100 per cent of your energy. This is the fun way to fitness.

this reason the styles you see in classes and clubs may vary considerably from one to another. The musical rhythms and the joy, enthusiasm and sheer physical energy of the dance unify the style.

The turns and swivels to be mastered in the dance will develop your muscular fitness and at the same time enhance your respiratory and cardiovascular fitness. Salsa demands a blend of precise footwork, responsiveness to rhythm and an extravagance of physical style. All of the above combine to challenge and develop your fitness and physical grace.

The best place to learn to salsa is at classes that provide you with the basic techniques and then go on to teach new steps and movements. Clubs will provide you with the opportunity to absorb the varying styles and steps of other dancers. Many classes are held in the early evening and then go on to a salsa club night – which gives you a good opportunity to put into practice the steps you have just learned in the class. Look in your local newspaper, library and dance schools for information on classes.

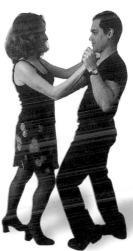

Look directly into your partner's eyes and keep as close as possible.

Before you move on to more advanced steps, you will need to learn how to hold your partner, make all the basic moves, how the arms move, what the legs are doing, and how to coordinate all of it into a smooth whole body rhythm. Further skills include how to turn at speed and how to move backward without losing technique or momentum.

Once this has become second nature, you can move on to more complex combinations of steps. If you have ever jived, you will recognize some of the turns, swirls and hand holds. Some other movements are taken directly from the tango and from many of the dances

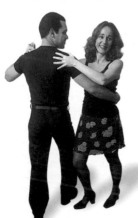

seen in the Dominican Republic, Colombia, Cuba and other Latin American countries – of course, with a little added spice.

Salsa is an undeniably sexy dance. You need

The turns, swirls and hand holds shown on these pages demonstrate the energy and emotional intensity of salsa. You will soon be moving backwards and turning at speed – and become thoroughly toned up in the process.

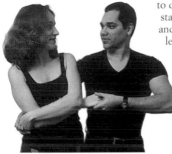

to develop your stamina, endurance and fitness on all levels to enjoy it fully. You also need to master the technique so that your and your partner's bodies are moving as one.

FACTFILE

Calories burnt per minute: 6.3

Works on: legs, arms, back, shoulders and buttocks

You need: clothing and shoes with some slip to make the dance moves properly. Trainers and other rubber-soled shoes are unsuitable

As you advance, you may wish to buy or make some of the typically colourful costumes that salsa dancers wear. For women, slinky, beaded, sparkling dresses in exotic colours, with high heels in a matching colour. For men, a brightly coloured shirt or waistcoat teamed with a colour-coordinated pair of trousers and shiny black shoes

The Alexander Technique

The Alexander Technique teaches you to be more aware of balance, posture and coordination while performing all sorts of everyday tasks (such as bending down, walking, sitting and standing). It teaches you to become conscious of previously unnoticed tensions throughout your body. These tensions, if unchecked, could lead to backache, headache, migraine, insomnia, arthritis, asthma, anxiety and depression.

As a child, you move naturally and flexibly, but as you grow up, bad habits are formed. You tend to slouch rather than hold yourself upright, and become lazy in the way you walk and sit, which can lead to rounded shoulders and a curved back. Poor posture impedes breathing and induces backache.

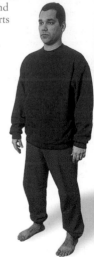

The Alexander Technique starts with the basics: how to stand and how to sit. Here you can see that the spine is taking as little stress as possible: the man stands with feet apart, shoulders relaxed, hands hanging loosely by his side. The neck is correctly aligned with the spine.

The Alexander Technique teaches you to unlearn these bad habits and revert to the posture you had as a child. It will help you to develop an awareness of your body and how it moves and increase your breathing and lung capacity, thereby improving circulation and strengthening the heart.

A qualified Alexander instructor will observe strains and tensions in your movements and through instruction and gentle manipulation will show you how to adopt the correct posture for your daily activities. Sessions are on a one to one basis and last between 30 and 45 minutes. The average number of lessons required is 20. It is especially useful to practise before and after exercise, so that your muscles and joints are as effectively warmed up as possible – you are then less likely to injure them.

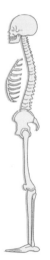

The two positions described below demonstrate quite clearly the effectiveness of this relatively simple but extremely beneficial form of exercise.

1 Put a small pile of books on the floor in a room that is warm and well

The principle behind the Alexander Technique is to establish a proper relationship of the head and neck to the rest of the body. This, in turn, will lead to the correct alignment of the vertebrae.

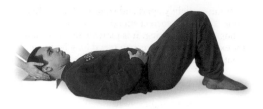

Lying in this position for about 20 minutes will show you the imbalances in your body and help you to regain some of the symmetry as well as relax, breathe properly and gain energy.

ventilated so that the muscles are relaxed. Lower yourself gently on to the floor, so that your head rests on the books. Your back should be on the floor and your knees bent so that they point up towards the ceiling. Your head should be in a comfortable position, your neck clear of the books. If the books are too low, your head will be pulled back, causing a strain on your throat. Your lower back will also be lifted off the floor, causing a strain on your spine. On the other hand, if the books are too high, your head will be pushed down, restricting your breathing (as your chin will be pressing into your larynx) and again your spine will take the strain.

2 When you sit down, take time to think about your posture. Don't just slump on to the chair. Your head should be poised and balanced on top of your spine. Your shoulders should be relaxed, your back and your bottom placed well to the back of the chair, with your knees slightly apart and your feet flat on the floor. This is the correct sitting position for leisure, for eating and for working. It is particularly important, for example, for people who spend long hours in front of a computer to sit correctly.

FACTFILE

Benefits: good posture, prevents spinal problems and overcomes breathing difficulties, alleviates stress and contributes to general well being

When sitting...

1 *Ensure that your neck and spine are in a straight line*

2 *Bend at the hips and knees.*

3 *Sit up straight: avoid slumping in the chair, leaning too far forward or over-arching your back.*

The bottom left posture is correct; the others are wrong.

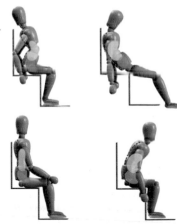

Yoga

Yoga is a philosophy that aims to achieve a state of physical, mental and spiritual well-being through the practice of postures, as well as through conscious relaxation and contemplation. It is a Hindu philosophy, and its meaning in Sanskrit is 'yoke' or 'union'. This refers to the union between the physical, mental and spiritual training that lies at the heart of yoga.

The postures, which are known as *asanas*, are practised slowly with concentration upon breathing, creating a sense of innermost peace and harmony.

A number of different systems of yoga are practised in the West, and so it is possible that no two teachers' classes will be quite the same. Hatha yoga is the best-known system in the West and concentrates on achieving physical and mental control and relaxation. Iyengar yoga, commonly practised in Britain, is a form of hatha yoga.

This elegant posture belies the fact the muscles of the buttocks and the hamstrings are fully extended and stretching beautifully. Yoga has much to offer the fitness enthusiast and it is well known for relieving anxiety and tension.

THE ASANAS

In the West, the physical aspect of yoga is widely practised. The postures (asanas) forming the basis of this type of yoga allow the body to relax as well as increasing its flexibility and overall fitness.

Developed over thousands of years, the asanas work on both the external body and internal organs. Each one has a particular purpose and they are often referred to by their Sanskrit names – for example, Tadasana (mountain pose), Halasana (plough) and Bhujangasana (cobra) – each easily identified with the respective pose.

Some are easy to assume, others need more practice before the muscles and limbs are supple enough. However, all involve two things:

1 A slow, deliberate stretching and releasing of the muscles. Each asana is done slowly and gracefully and held

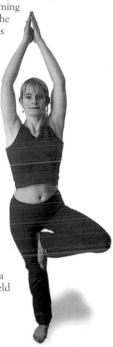

The Vrksasana (tree). As you start to develop better balance through muscular strength, you will be able to achieve the more graceful yoga postures.

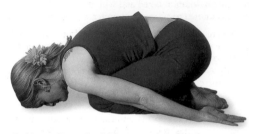

Garbhasana (pose of a child) is a tremendously relaxing and revitalizing posture. Hold it for a couple of minutes and be sure to uncurl yourself slowly.

for a few minutes, avoiding all strain and allowing you to develop an awareness of your physical body and internal and external tensions.

2 Correct breathing is an integral part of yoga. You are encouraged to breathe more deeply and fully, filling the chest and the abdomen with each breath. The breath is exhaled slowly from deep in the diaphragm. Becoming more conscious of your breathing allows you to release the physical tension throughout your body.

Balance is another key aspect. The sequence of postures complement each other to provide a work-out for the entire body. For example, a bend to one side will be followed by a bend to the other, a forward bend will be counterposed with a backward bend.

The postures reduce stress, making you sleep better and

leaving you calm, relaxed and with an untroubled mind. Yoga is known to promote an inner and outer harmony.

There are about 80 principal postures, but most people practise only a small number of these. It is important to have a qualified teacher so that you learn the asanas exactly as they should be performed and breathe in and out at the correct moment. A class will last an hour to an hour and a half and you will generally be taken through 10–15 postures. It is important to begin with warm-up exercises and to end the yoga session with at least ten minutes' relaxation. As classes vary from teacher to teacher, it is worthwhile trying out a few to find the one that is right for you. You will find classes at nearly all adult education institutes and at many health clubs (see Useful addresses).

If you suffer from high blood pressure, back trouble or if you are pregnant, speak to a qualified teacher about what you can do. The postures can be modified.

FACTFILE

Benefits: tones up muscles, increases suppleness and flexibility, develops strength and dexterity, improves the circulation, works on internal bodily functions, relieves stress and increases mental clarity and control

Complementary exercises: walking, swimming, jogging, running

The martial arts

The Eastern systems of physical and mental training, known collectively as the martial arts are used for self-understanding, expression through movement and self-defence. The systems share common aims and are often interrelated. Examples include the Japanese arts of aikido, judo, jujitsu, karate and kendo, the Chinese arts of t'ai chi ch'uan and kung fu (of which there are many forms) and tae kwon do (from Korea).

Each martial art has a different style. Karate, tae kwon do and many forms of kung fu rely mainly on punches, kicks and blocks, whereas judo and jujitsu rely on throws and holds using balance as a primary force. Aikido teaches the student to use the attacker's aggression and momentum against him/her. The opponent's joints (wrist, elbow and shoulder) and pressure points are used in applying techniques and moves.

Judo practitioners rely on balance. Having unbalanced your opponent you can now move in for a throw.

Weapons are also involved. Kendo uses the Japanese sword (katana and bokken); aikido, the sword and staff (bo); and karate, the rice flail (nunchuku). For certain Japanese arts, a 'gi' (uniform) must be worn. This comprises loose trousers, jacket and belt.

The martial arts are intended to be used in times of self-defence, and only when confrontation is unavoidable. The serious student is actively encouraged to learn the philosophy behind the art, making a commitment to long-term study.

Classes, which are usually held once or twice a week, often start with a brief meditation and warm-up exercises. The level of experience gained is measured by the colour of belt the practitioner wears; from white (beginner) to black (expert). In between, there are many different levels.

Practice increases flexibility, strength, dexterity, speed, agility, balance and encourages mental clarity and control. All martial arts should be practised under the direct supervision of a qualified instructor.

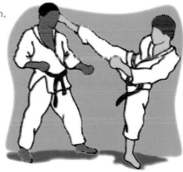

Karate practitioners use punches and kicks to strike their opponent. Good balance and suppleness are required.

T'ai chi

This gentle, meditative system of exercises, designed to challenge both the body and the mind, has been practised in the Far East for many years. It has been a common sight for decades to see large groups of people in parks and other large public spaces (even car parks) in mainland China and in Hong Kong practising the movements of t'ai chi, and it is becoming increasingly popular in the West.

T'ai chi consists of a system of gentle, circular movements and positions (rather like swimming in the air) that aim to exercise the muscles, unify body and

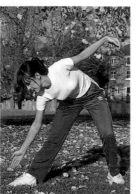

mind and encourage an even flow of 'chi' (inner energy) through the body – all of which results in an all-round increase in health and vitality. T'ai chi is suitable for almost everyone since there is little or no risk of injury and the meditative quality of the system has

With your weight on your bent left leg and your right leg straight, extend your right arm over your right leg and your left arm back over your shoulder.

tremendous appeal for those who are not attracted to more aggressive or competitive forms of exercise. It can also be used effectively as a complement to more vigorous, physical exercises, particularly as a way to relieve any muscular tension.

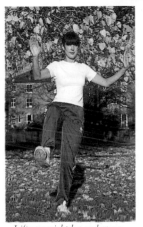

Lift your right leg and move your left hand up. Turn your right palm upward and away from you.

T'ai chi means Supreme Ultimate Power and the system is believed to express the blending of the eternal and the temporal, heaven and earth. As an exercise system, it has the potential to improve muscle tone, to control the movements of the body and is believed to strengthen the gastrointestinal tract, therefore aiding elimination of waste matter. In common with other types of exercise, it also relieves stress and anxiety. T'ai chi deepens the breathing and so is believed to increase oxygen to the bloodstream, opening the blood vessels and allowing the heart to function more smoothly. Balance and physical coordination are improved through rigorously carrying

Place your right foot on the ground, one step behind your left foot. Push your right hand forward, palm forward and fingers up. Lower your left elbow until your hand is near your waist.

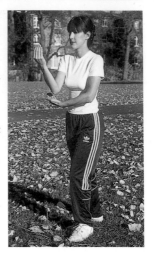

out the exercises and many people find that it relieves arthritis, promotes agility and stamina and gives relief from pain.

The short form of t'ai chi consists of 37 different movements (some illustrated here) that can be performed in about 7 to 10 minutes. The long form of the same movements would take at least 20 minutes, if not more. One movement flows rhythmically into the next. In all there are 128 different movements to be learned, each one based on the natural movements found in nature – for example, the wind, birds in flight, and the sea. The practice of the movements is said to maintain a state of natural flow by stabilizing the body's fluctuating energies of yin and yang – opposing and complementary forces that reflect the ceaseless ebb and flow of life.

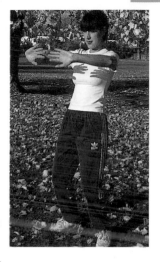

Stand relaxed, knees slightly bent. Bend your elbows slightly and lift your arms to shoulder height in front of you, hands and fingers to be horizontal and relaxed.

For maximum respiratory benefit, consider practising t'ai chi in the open air. Breathe in fully and naturally from your abdomen and make your movements with careful deliberateness and with slow, flowing continuity. Concentrate on your movements to achieve total mental and physical relaxation.

Classes are widely available at evening institutes, health clubs and centres (see Useful addresses).

FACTFILE

Benefits: good for muscular tone, overall flexibility, breathing, relieving stress; concentration, self-awareness and control of mind and body

HEALTHY MIND, HEALTHY BODY

The feel-good factor

Anyone who has ever exercised on a regular basis will testify to the feel-good quality that results. Exercise and sport have the power to refresh the mind, blow away the cobwebs, tone up the circulation, bring a bloom to the skin, strengthen the muscles, improve the posture and deepen the breathing.

Regular and sustained physical exercise improves concentration and memory while also enhancing your psychological well-being. This aids the enjoyment of exercise and sport and will quite quickly encourage adherence to an exercise programme. It is an upward spiral once you start using your body.

So well documented are the benefits of exercise for psychological health and well-being that the NHS now gives some people on low income free vouchers to enable them to attend leisure centres so that they may swim and undertake forms of exercise.

WHAT HAPPENS TO THE BRAIN

One of the reasons why exercise has such a profound psychological effect on well-being lies in the fact that levels of certain chemicals in the brain, known as

DON'TS

Beware of dehydration – remember to drink water before and after exercise

Don't exercise in sub-zero temperatures nor in unusually hot weather

Don't exercise when you are ill – if you have a cold, wait until you are fully recovered before beginning with very light exercise. Gradually build up again over a 2-week period. If your illness is more serious, seek medical advice before returning to exercise

endorphins, increase during exercise. Endorphins have been called the feel-good hormones. They are responsible for exerting physiological and psychological effects. They are the same hormones that are released during and after lovemaking.

This chemical process may explain why some people become dependent on regular exercise for their well-being and feel unwell and deprived if for any reason they are unable to exercise. The process also explains how people can enjoy, not merely tolerate, really strenuous exercise such as endurance running as endorphins also act as painkillers and heighten pleasure. You only have to look at the faces of marathon runners to see the euphoria. This is caused not just by their sense of achievement but also by the chemical changes taking place in the body. They simply Feel Good.

FITNESS FIGHTS FATIGUE

It may seem hard after a full day's work to go for a long walk, to play a game of squash or to go to the local pool to swim 25 lengths. However, it is a fact that you will feel better for doing this than if you go home, have supper and lie around dozing and watching TV or reading a book.

After you have made the initial effort to exercise, you may be surprised to find that your heart will be pumping more efficiently, your breathing will deepen, your muscles will obtain the freshly oxygenated blood more effectively – and you will achieve that all-important release of endorphins. Your posture and self-confidence will also improve – and this carries through to the next day as well. In the meantime, exercise usually provides a better quality of sleep than if you had not exercised.

The benefits of regular exercise will be even greater if you can fit in a 20- or 30-minute session in the morning rather than in the evening. Now you will be set up for the demands of the day with a higher metabolic rate and an increased energy level.

MENTAL BENEFITS OF EXERCISE

Doctors, psychiatrists and psychologists, and many other healthcare professionals now recognize the benefits of exercise. It is known that regular and sustained exercise helps to:

• Allay anxiety and fight off depression

- Relieve physical and mental stresses and tensions
- Improve concentration and memory
- Give you the opportunity to think through problems and dilemmas
- Improve your quality of sleep, thus enabling you to cope better with the demands of the following day
- Enhance your sense of having control over your life
- Increase your self-confidence and self-esteem
- Encourage you to think positively about all the areas of your life – your work, home and family and your life as an individual person

Remember that fitness fights fatigue – so take control of your life!

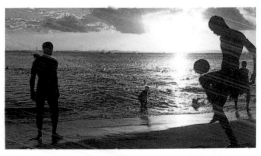

Walking and swimming are thought to be the two best possible means of exercise and relaxation.

Chilling out

All of us need to relax fully and consciously – on a
regular basis. Conscious relaxation involves something
more refreshing than simply dozing in front of a warm
fire. True relaxation should leave you feeling refreshed
and invigorated rather than sluggish. While you relax,
try to empty your mind of thoughts, to focus upon a
nothingness and achieve a trance-like state. When you
are feeling fully relaxed, your heart rate will decrease,
your eyelids may feel heavy, and you may feel slightly
chilly, so have a sweater handy.

Modern life proves stressful for many of us and there is
no doubt that the pace of life, particularly at work, has
increased considerably towards the end of the 20th
century. Many of us are faced with a gruelling schedule
of getting up, getting the children up and dressed,
getting ready for work, taking the children to school,
doing a full day's work, preparing the supper ... and
there is no let-up.

WHEN DO YOU FIND A FEW FREE
MOMENTS FOR YOURSELF?

- All you need is at least 15 minutes a day in which to
  achieve a fully relaxed state. More would of course be
  beneficial.

- Can you, for example, use part of your lunch hour for
  one of the forms of relaxation listed below?

- Can you get up half an hour earlier in the morning in order to devote half an hour to a relaxation technique?
- You may find it easier to devote an hour at the weekend to one of the relaxation methods, and concentrate on physical exercise and your everyday lifestyle during the week.

Remember, chilling out is an essential part of keeping fit: its importance cannot be overemphasized.

Some of the activities we do for the purpose of keeping fit can also be done, much more slowly and with a less goal-oriented attitude, for the purpose of relaxation. For example, you can walk at a vigorous speed, even at racewalking speed, to increase maximum fitness. But you can also go for a stroll in order to get some fresh air into your lungs and relax.

Warm-up, cool down and stretch 'n' tone exercises can also be used as part of your relaxation programme. These exercises can now be regarded as a relaxation therapy for your body and mind, and needn't be seen exclusively in terms of improving fitness. The repetitive nature of these exercises makes them perfect for freeing the mind of everyday concerns and for allowing your thoughts to wander.

RELAXATION TECHNIQUES

As you will see, some of the relaxation techniques that are described below are active methods of relaxation,

while others are more passive. Choose whichever
appeals to you the most.

MEDITATION

Meditation can induce a state of total relaxation, inner
peace and harmony and increase your mental, physical
and spiritual awareness. Although it is often associated
with world religions such as Buddhism, a non-religious
style of meditation has emerged in the West in recent
years and is widely practised. Meditation can increase
your energy levels, improve your concentration and
blood circulation, release muscular tension and give
relief from pain. The deep relaxation and increased
mental clarity that meditation brings also relieve stress.

Techniques include focusing on a specific object,
emptying the mind of all thoughts or concentrating
solely on the body. You can have one-to-one instruction,
or a class (30–60 minutes) or teach yourself to meditate.

How to meditate

• Find a quiet comfortable environment.

• Lie on your back on the floor with the palms of your
  hands outstretched and facing upward. Have a
  cushion to place under your neck/head. Make sure
  your neck is in a comfortable position.

• Close your eyes.

• Consciously relax every part of your body, one part at
  a time, bit by bit.

• Concentrate on your feet and toes. Let them relax.

- Now direct your thoughts to your legs, concentrating on relaxing first your calves and then your thighs.
- Is your spine supple and relaxed, are your shoulders lying flat to the floor and in an opened-out position?
- Let your arms go, and now relax your wrists and hands.
- Concentrate on your breathing. Feel your abdominal muscles work as your breathing deepens and slows.
- Let your mind float freely. Try not to think about anything in particular.
- Remain like this for up to 20 minutes.
- Get up slowly and stretch out your limbs, one by one, and your back.

VISUALIZATION

Focusing on positive images and desired outcomes to specific situations allows you to cope with problems and fulfil potential. Visualization is used as a relaxation therapy, often in conjunction with psychotherapy and hypnotherapy. You can do it alone, on a one-to-one basis or in a class (lasting approximately 30–60 minutes).

How to visualize

- Sit in a comfortable chair or lie on your back on the floor.
- Close your eyes.
- Choose a scene that spells peace and tranquillity to you, for example, a seascape that you know well. What matters is that its message is quiet and relaxing.

- Focus on this scene – the general composition and all the detail – for up to 20 minutes.
- Allow yourself to be drawn into the picture of your choice and to exclude everything else around you.

Relax and visualize yourself as powerful, fit, supple and confident. Repeat these affirmations to yourself: 'I am fit and healthy. Peak fitness is my goal'.

YOGA

See pp 152–155.

MASSAGE

Aromatherapy massage is one of the most delicious, sensual and luxurious relaxation treatments available. Special care is taken in blending essential oils together for each individual. Oils are extracted from the roots, flowers, leaves and stalks of plants. Each oil has its own fragrance, therapeutic properties and medicinal qualities. During massage, the oils are absorbed into the pores of the skin and inhaled through the nose. Aromatherapy massage will vary from practitioner to practitioner, but is largely based on the Swedish style where long, slow, gentle massage strokes are used. Massage is believed to help ease tight muscles, improve circulation and remove waste matter from the body. It also helps to release unwanted nervous tension stored up in muscles. Finally, it promotes a general feeling of well-being. Have a professional massage or teach yourself (books and classes are widely available).

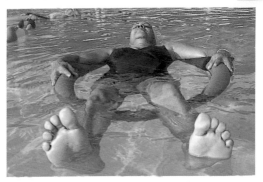

Many forms of hydrotherapy are energizing and invigorating.

HYDROTHERAPY

'Hydro' (meaning water) therapy is any form of water therapy. Water, in its various forms, is able to influence blood flow. It may be used internally and externally, hot or cold, as liquid, steam or ice, to cleanse, revitalize, restore and maintain health. Cold water stimulates, restricts blood flow, reduces inflammation and sends more blood to the organs. Hot water dilates blood vessels, reduces blood pressure and increases the blood flow to muscles and skin. Water treatments include:

• High-powered jets to stimulate circulation

• Sea water jets, wraps and baths to cleanse and relax

- Compresses, water-soaked towels applied to the body to ease stiff muscles, reduce inflammation
- Steam baths and saunas to cleanse and relieve water retention

Hydrotherapy is available at health farms and health clubs or your GP may recommend a physiotherapist who uses it.

THE ALEXANDER TECHNIQUE

See pp 148–151

COLOUR THERAPY

It is widely accepted that colour affects our moods and feelings. Research has shown, for example, that yellow, orange or red will increase our learning ability and that blue and black are the most calming of all colours. Colour therapists concentrate on providing you with the colours that they perceive you need. If you are suffering from stress and anxiety, your therapist will focus on relaxing colours for you. Treatment is administered either through a colour therapy instrument, which uses stained glass for filters, or through contact healing with the hands (see Useful addresses).

SELF-HYPNOSIS

Hypnosis is a distinct level of consciousness between waking and deep sleep, in which you experience an altered state of reality, a state of total relaxation. When you are truly hypnotized, you bypass the conscious part of the brain to access the subconscious. You will remain open to suggestion and in this way hypnosis can be used to attain inner calm and relaxation, but also to allay any anxieties and fears. Ideally, you should see a professional hypnotherapist to learn the techniques of self-hypnosis, then practise at home.

The body needs to rest and repair itself, and so does the mind. It is exercise and relaxation in combination that produce true psychological calm. The psychological benefits of conscious relaxation will spill over into your enjoyment of physical exercise. Chill Out!

COMMON MISCONCEPTIONS

- Alcohol. Many people drink to relax themselves, but alcohol works firstly as a stimulant and then as a depressant, which is not genuinely relaxing.

- Smoking. Despite smokers' claims that a cigarette calms the nerves, nicotine in fact only affords a brief respite (about 20 minutes) from the craving for more nicotine.

- TV. The couch potato habit is an easy one to acquire but a harder one to shake off. It is relaxing in the short term, but it is entirely passive and does not relax you in the same way as the Chilling Out techniques do.

Optimum vitality

We can achieve optimum vitality by looking at the areas of our lives listed below. The first three of these areas have already been covered in this book:

- Diet – for nutrition
- Exercise – for fitness
- Relaxation – for health
- Sleep – of good quality
- Health – physical and mental
- Freedom from stress and problems
- An enjoyable life – doing some of the things you like doing some of the time
- Developing your confidence and self-esteem
- Thinking positively – training yourself into a positive thinking style

Let's look at the remaining six areas that have not been fully covered.

SLEEP

We all know how insistent the urge to sleep can be and how miserable you can feel if you resist that urge to sleep. Regular sleep is essential for your physical and mental well-being. Sleep is a period of restoration, a time during which certain biological and mental processes take place.

There are two types of sleep: REM (rapid eye movement sleep), which is when most dreaming occurs and NREM (non-REM sleep), which is dreamless. During NREM, the body repairs and regenerates itself, whereas in REM, dreams are thought to help us sort out our emotional problems. Most people need about 7–8 hours' sleep a night, although it varies from person to person and decreases with age. To get a good night's sleep:

- Avoid stimulants such as coffee last thing at night
- Do some form of aerobic exercise in the day
- Make sure your bedroom is well-ventilated
- Go to bed at a regular time
- Slow down mental activity before bed; try to do some breathing and relaxation exercises (see pp 24–27).

HEALTH

For optimum vitality, take a critical look at your state of health. Do you have unresolved medical problems that you know you should discuss with your doctor? If so, make the appointment now. Dental appointments and optometry tests are also vitally important, not only for the sake of your teeth and eyesight but also for your general health. Some diseases are diagnosed first through checking the eyes.

Optimum vitality and health will show itself in the condition of your gums, eyes, hair and skin. A slightly greyish pallor could be indicative of a lack of fresh air, poor health and/or a lack of fitness generally.

Good health includes mental health. One in four of us will suffer at some time in our life from some sort of mental illness. Depression, for example, is widespread and often goes unrecognized, finding its outlet in drinking to excess, marital rows and destructive behaviour. If you feel 'not quite yourself', don't hesitate to seek help from your family doctor.

FREEDOM FROM STRESS

Some stress in your life is not necessarily a bad thing: it is a normal response to a challenge and can actually be very stimulating. However, too much stress, particularly of the emotional variety, can be harmful to both your physical and mental well-being. It is associated with high blood pressure and muscular tension, can cause long-term fatigue and may erode your overall fitness and sense of well-being.

If you are feeling too stressed:

- Sit down and make a list of the things that are worrying you. Looking at problems one by one can make them seem a lot less intimidating

- Try to put things into perspective – does it really matter if you don't do something?

- Are there practical ways of changing what is causing the stress? A small change can make a big difference

- Are you creating stress for yourself? Have you taken on too much? Could you do things in a different way?

- Talk to your partner, a friend or colleague

- Try to make some quiet time for yourself every day
- Do regular exercise – it's a good stress reliever

ENJOYING YOUR LIFE

You have your working life, your family life and your private life as an individual. Do you personally have something to look forward to that is specially for you rather than for your friends, your family, your children or your work? An essential part of enjoying life is learning how to put yourself first.

Make a list of the activities you really enjoy and work out how much time a week you actually spend on those activities. Many of us discover that it is not very much time at all. Remember, it is your life.

Make time for yourself – do things you find enjoyable and relaxing.

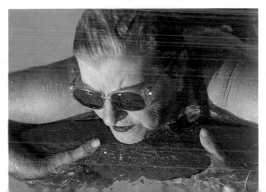

DEVELOPING SELF-BELIEF

Many people find that they can begin to develop their confidence and self-esteem through taking control of their lives. Eating properly, exercising and resolving long-term problems are all integral parts of this process.

All of us need to learn that we have the right to say 'No' in order to avoid becoming overloaded with work or family commitments. It takes self-esteem, and a realization of your worth as a person, to be able to say 'No' without worrying that others will think less of you.

THINK POSITIVELY

There is always more than one way of viewing things in life. Do you try to see the positive aspects of a situation or a person? This is an important consideration for your general vitality. The more positively you think, the more positively you are likely to be regarded. It is a real truth that what you give out is what you get back.

Do you sometimes go out of your way to please someone, to wish them well for a particular event, to enquire and care about their well-being?

Can you say that you are not overly critical and intolerant of others? Compassion and empathy are important aspects of thinking positively about other people.

Take a good look at the elements of your life and see how much good there is in it.

Finally, to develop your full vitality and vigour, take the time now and then to stop and stand back. Try to avoid

becoming wrapped up in the demands of everyday life.
Because that is what they are – everyday demands. They
will continue, day after day. Don't put exercising for
fitness and yourself on the back burner while you just sort
this and then sort that out. Think of Yourself and Keep
Fit for Life: it will benefit you and everyone around you.

*Putting yourself to the challenge and winning through is the
ultimate achievement, a testament to the work that you have put
in to achieve peak fitness. Vitality, invigoration and feeling good
are what fitness is all about.*

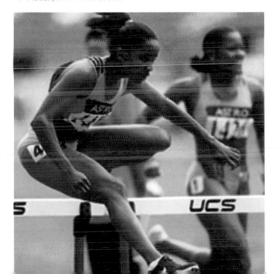

USEFUL ADDRESSES

Amateur Boxing Association of England Ltd
Crystal Palace National
Sports Centre
London SE19 2BB
T: 0181–778 0251

Amateur Rowing Association
6 Lower Mall
London W6 9DJ
T: 0181–748 3632

Amateur Swimming Association
Harold Fern House
Derby Square
Loughborough
Leicester LE11 5AL
T: 01509–618 700

Association of British Riding Schools
Queen's Chambers
38–40 Queen Street
Penzance
Cornwall TR18 4BH
T: 01736–369 440

British Athletics Association
Centres nationwide. Contact
your local sport centre.

British Cycling Federation
National Cycling Centre
Stuart Street
Manchester M11 4DQ
T: 0161–230 2301

British Gymnastics
Ford Hall
Lilleshall National Sports
Centre
Near Newport
Shropshire TF10 9NB
T: 01952–820 330

British Horse Society
Stoneleigh Deer Park
Kenilworth
Warwickshire CV8 2XZ
T: 01926–707 700

International Badminton Federation
Manor Park Place
Rutherford Way
Cheltenham
Gloucestershire GL51 9TU
T: 01242–234 904

International Tennis Federation
Bank Lane

Roehampton
London SW15 5XZ
T: 0181–878 6464

**The Lawn Tennis
Association**
Head Office
Queen's Club
West Kensington
London W14 9EG
T: 0171–381 7000

Quit for Life
Health Research Centre
Middlesex University
Queensway
Enfield EN3 4SF
Middlesex
T: 0181–362 5558

Ramblers' Association
1/5 Wandsworth Road
London SW8 2XX
T: 0171–339 8500

**The Royal and Ancient
Golf Club of St Andrews**
St Andrews
Fife KY16 9JD
Scotland
T: 01334–472 112

World Squash Federation
6 Havelock Road
Hastings
East Sussex TN34 1BP
T: 01424–429 245

Aromatherapy

Aromatherapy massage is
offered by health farms and
clubs, sports centres and
beauty clinics. Professional
aromatherapists should have
attended an accredited college.
To obtain a copy of a list of
accredited therapists write to:
PO Box 52
Market Harborough
Leicester LE16 8ZX

Aromatherapy Trade Council
3 Latymer Close
Braybrooke
Market Harborough
Leicestershire LE16 8LN
T: 01858–465 731

Colour Therapy

Association of Colour Therapists
c/o ICM
21 Portland Place
London W1 3AS

Hygeia Studios Ltd
Colour Teaching Research
Brook House
Hampton Hill
Avening
Tetbury
Gloucestershire GL8 8NS
T: 01453–832 150

The International Association for Colour Therapy
73 Elm Bank Gardens
London SW13 0NX

Hydrotherapy

Most health spas offer some form of hydrotherapy. Many naturopaths are highly skilled in hydrotherapy.

The British College of Naturopathy and Osteopathy
Frazer House
6 Netherhall Gardens
London NW3 5RR
T: 0171–435 6464

Hypnotherapy

British Hypnotherapy Association
67 Upper Berkeley Street
London W1H 7DH
T: 0171–723 4443

The National College of Hypnosis and Psychotherapy
12 Cross Street
Nelson
Lancashire BB9 7EN
T: 01282–699 378

Martial arts

British Council for Chinese Martial Arts
c/o 110 Frensham Drive
Popular Farm
Nuneaton
Warwickshire CV10 9QL
T: 01203–394 642

European Wushu Federation
11 Lucas Close
Yatchley
Camberly GU17 7JO

Meditation

Classes are held by meditation schools and are often advertised in libraries and newspapers.

**Friends of the Western
Buddhist Order**
London Buddhist Centre
51 Roman Road
London E2 0HU
T: 0181-981 1225

School of Meditation
158 Holland Park Avenue
London W11 4UH
T: 0171-603 6116

Transcendental Meditation
Freepost
London SW1P 4YY
T: 0990-143 733

Relaxation and breathing

**The Stress Management
Training Institute**
Foxhills
30 Victoria Avenue
Shanklin
Isle of Wight PO37 6LS
T: 01983-868 166

T'ai chi
Classes advertised in local
libraries, health clubs,
community centres and
newspapers.

**T'ai chi Union
for Great Britain**
23 Oakwood Avenue
Mitcham
Surrey CR4 3DQ

Visualization
**UK Council for
Psychotherapy**
167-69 Great Portland Street
London W1N 5FB
T: 0171-436 3002

Yoga
Classes advertised in local
libraries, health clubs,
community centres and
newspapers.

**The International
Yoga School**
The Kevala Centre
Hunsdon Road
Torquay
Devon TQ1 1QB
T: 01803-215 678

Yoga Therapy Centre
The Royal London
Homeopathic Hospital
60 Great Ormond Street
London WC1N 3HR
T: 0171-419 7195

INDEX

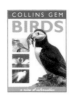
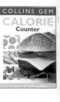